knee pain

The Self-Help Guide

by John Garrett, M.D.
& Bob Reznik, M.B.A.

Foreword by Richard Steadman, M.D.

New Harbinger Publications, Inc.

Publisher's Note

This publication is designed to provide accurate and authoritative information in regard to the subject matter covered. It is sold with the understanding that the publisher is not engaged in rendering psychological, financial, legal, or other professional services. If expert assistance or counseling is needed, the services of a competent professional should be sought.

Distributed in the U.S.A. by Publishers Group West; in Canada by Raincoast Books; in Great Britain by Airlift Book Company, Ltd.; in South Africa by Real Books, Ltd.; in Australia by Boobook; and in New Zealand by Tandem Press.

Published by New Harbinger Publications, Inc.
5674 Shattuck Avenue
Oakland, CA 94609

Copyright © 2000 by   Prizm Development, Inc.
181 Grand Ave, Suite 212
Southlake, TX 76092

Photography: Paul Buck, Bob Reznik
Stock photography sources: Corbis, Photodisc, Digital Stock
Book design: Bob Reznik
Cover design: Cary Terry
Cover photos: Paul Buck, John Reznik
Illustrations: Nucleus Communications
Editorial Assistant: Christi Beard
Edited by: Lorna Garano

Library of Congress Catalog Card Number: 99-75289
ISBN 1-57224-194-2 Paperback

Printed in the United States of America

New Harbinger Publications' Web site address: www.newharbinger.com.

02   01   00

10   9   8   7   6   5   4   3   2   1

First printing

To my wife Wendy, and my three sons, John, Mark, and Andrew.
Thanks for your patience during the long evenings and weekends
spent on this book. Hey, I'm ready now. Let's play tennis.
— Bob Reznik, MBA

To our wives,
Joy Garrett and Gay Steadman,
for their encouragement and inspiration.
— John Garrett, M.D. & Richard Steadman, M.D.

Knee Pain: The Self-Help Guide
CONTENTS

Acknowledgments xi
Forward xiii

Introduction

About Self-Help 1

Part 1: About Knees

Chapter 1

Everything You Need to Know about Knees 5
  Who Can Benefit from This Book? 7
  Staying Active as You Age 8
  Just How Long Can the Original Parts Last? 8
  Your Current Choices Will Affect Your Retirement 10
  Choosing to Stay Active 10
  The Knee is the Crux, or the Crutch of It All 11
  How We Live Can Affect Our Knees 12
  How This Book Can Help Your Knee Problem 13
  Ask Questions, Be Informed, and Seek out the Best Quality Care 14
  Where Does Knee Pain Come From? 15
  The Four Most Common Knee Problems 16
  Treatment of Knee Pain: Where We've Been 17
  Treatment of Knee Pain: Where We Are Now 18
  Treatment of Knee Pain: Where We Are Going in the Next Century 19
  Diagnosing Knee Problems 20

Chapter 2

Anatomy Lesson 23
  Bone Up on Your Knee Knowledge 24
  Articular Cartilage 26
  Meet the Meniscus 27
  What are "Ligaments"? 29
  Tendons, Muscles, Nerves, Blood Vessels in the Knees 32

Part 2: Knee Pain and Its Causes

Chapter 3

What Causes Knee Pain? 37
    Strains, Sprains, and Tears 38
    What is Inflammation? 39
    Pain from Meniscus Tears 40
    Chondromalacia 41
    Ligament Problems 42
    The Torn ACL Ligament 43
    Other Ligament Tears 43
    Tendon Trouble 45
    Arthritis 46
    Rheumatoid Arthritis 48
    Crystalline Arthritis 48
    A Crack or Out of Whack? 49
    Dislocation 51
    Knee Problems That Affect Kids 51
    Communicating with Kids 56
    Pre-Patellar Bursitis 57
    Plica Syndrome 58
    Coming up Next 58

Chapter 4

Diagnosing Knee Pain: What Do Various Symptoms Mean? 61
    Which Symptoms are Significant? 61
    Fractures 62
    Ligament Tears 63
    Tendon Problems 64
    Meniscal Damage 64
    Joint Problems 65
    How a Doctor Diagnoses Knee Problems 66
    Time for a Visit to the Knee Doctor 75
    Acute Knee Pain: Flow Chart for Self-Diagnosis 82
    Some Common Questions 88

Part 3: Treatment

Chapter 5

How You Can Treat Some Knee Problems Without Surgery 93
  About Severity of Tears, and the Ability of Certain Ligaments
  to Heal on their Own 94
  Anti-Inflammatories and Medicating Yourself 95
  Do It Yourself Physical Therapy 97
  Orthotics and Braces 98
  About Knee Braces and Support Wraps 99
  Dieting to Reduce Knee Pain 103
  Are You Overweight? 106
  The Role of Food 106
  Dietary Supplements 107
  Vitamins and Their Effect on Our Bodies 115
  What about Alternative Medicine for Knee Problems? 116
  Herbs: A Natural Medicine 119
  Alternative Treatments for Knee Pain 121
  A Final Note about Sports Supplements 130

Chapter 6

Exercises to Relieve Knee Pain 131
  Before You Get Started on Your Knee Exercises 133
  How Chapter 6 and Chapter 9 Exercises Differ 134

Chapter 7

When Surgery Must Be Considered 155
  Repair of the Torn Anterior Cruciate Ligament 156
  Repairing the Permanently Damaged Knee Joint
  with Total Knee Joint Replacement 167
  The Total Knee Joint Replacement Surgery 174
  Knee Implant Surgery: The Second Time Around 184
  Advances in Knee Treatment coming in the Next Ten Years 184
  Joint Surface Replacement 185
  Transplantation of Segments of a Joint Surface 186
  Bowed Legs and Arthritis 188

Part 4: Staying Informed and Injury-Free

Chapter 8

Finding the Best Knee Surgeon 191
Step 1: Board Certification 193
Step 2: Look for High Volume, Practice Specialization,
and Fellowship Training 194
Step 3: Designation as a Knee Center of Excellence by a
Health Plan or Employer 196
Step 4: Check Any Available Lists and Subsets 197
Step 5: Call Any Policing Organizations for Information
on Complaints or Malpractice Claims 199
Step 6: Be Willing to Travel for the Best Knee Doctor 199
Step 7: Access the Internet 202

Chapter 9

How to Prevent Knee Pain 203
Preventing Knee Injury from Skiing 204
Basketball 209
Football 210
Soccer 211
Golf 211
Tennis and Other Racquet Sports 212
Running and Jogging 213
Walking 214
Biking 214
Swimming 215
Footgear for Sports 215
Knee Braces for Sports 216
Preventing Knee Injuries in Kids 216
Exercises That Make the Knee Injury-Resistant 218

Chapter 10

How to Use the Internet to the Benefit of Your Knees 229
Search Engines 230
Checking Up on Doctors 233
General Resource Sites on the Internet 232
Using the Internet to Find a Knee Doctor 232
Our Favorite Orthopedic Sites 236

Our Favorite General Health Sites *239*
Web sites for Researching Alternative Medicine *243*
Web sites for Nutrition and Weight Management *243*
Reviewing a Doctor's Web site *243*
A Final Cautionary Not about Quackery on the Internet *244*

References *246*
INDEX *247*

ACKNOWLEDGMENTS

For their help in the therapy section of this book,
our appreciation goes to:

Mr. Shawn McEnroe
Physical Therapist at Steadman-Hawkins Clinic
Vail, Colorado

Ms. Jeri Cruse
Physical Therapist for the physicians at Resurgens Orthopaedics
Atlanta, Georgia

by
Richard Steadman, M.D.

Each year at the Steadman-Hawkins Clinic, we see a variety of knee problems come through our doors. Torn ligaments, strained tendons, degenerative arthritis, damaged cartilage, torn menisci—we've treated them all.

Even though these knee pain sufferers come to us with a range of problems, they all have one thing in common: an intense desire to be mobile again so they can walk, run, perform, or compete as they did in the past.

We often take for granted the smooth, normal function of our legs. Sadly, good knee health is sometimes appreciated only after it has deteriorated.

Fortunately, many of those who come to Vail for consultation will go home successfully treated and more active than they previously were. Unfortunately, some knee pain sufferers, who have developed arthritis will need to come to grips with the fact that this disease is a life changing one. There is no miracle which will restore an arthritic joint to the smooth functioning machine it was in its youth.

However, by taking an organized approach and choosing the correct treatment options, it is usually possible to return the arthritis sufferer to an acceptable and satisfying form of exercise.

Knee Pain: The Self-Help Guide will provide general information to those suffering from knee pain. It should be considered a handbook for those seeking healthier knees.

For others with degenerative joint problems who may have to accept some permanent compromise, this book offers suggestions for regaining a level of physical activity by finding a pain-free movement zone. With special exercises, this zone can be expanded slightly, so more pain-free activity is possible than before.

What Are the Patient's Expectations?

My first task as a physician is to evaluate the goals and expectations of each patient, based on the severity of his or her knee problem. An elite skier might *expect* to return from injury to competition in giant slalom on the U.S. Ski Team.

On the other hand, a middle-aged arthritis sufferer may wish to simply walk a mile three times a week to stay physically fit. In both cases, the two things that will influence the achievement of either goal will be the type of problem each patient has, and his or her motivation to rehabilitate a painful knee to the strength level of a healthy one.

Based on my experience, a competitive and successful professional athlete who sustains a knee injury will have a good chance of full recovery from most simple knee problems. This patient has already demonstrated toughness and determination in achieving a professional goal.

The amateur athlete, on the other hand, may have to adjust his or her expectations to coincide with the level of effort brought to the rehabilitation process.

Knee pain can be a problem that begins in middle age. Although many of our patients are sports professionals, we also see middle-aged athletes who are frustrated because their knees will no longer function painlessly. To add insult to injury, some of these weekend warriors have gradually added extra pounds to their frames.

This naturally places even greater stress on knee joints, and increases the risk of injury. Losing the excess weight could improve knee health for these people, but unfortunately, they are not reminded of this.

A professional athlete will sometimes risk injury because money and fame are strong motivators, and his livelihood may depend upon it. The recreational athlete with a painful knee usually has a mechanical problem that can be solved, but it takes good advice, time, and hard work to return to full activity. It is clear that professional and amateur must travel the same road to recovery.

Learning from Others in Gaining Motivation

Part of our success with professional athletes is related to the examples set by others faced with potentially career-ending injuries. Their recoveries and subsequent athletic victories provide the strong medicines of hope and encouragement to our patients.

When Olympic skier, Phil Mahre, shattered his ankle in 1979, many felt he would be lucky to ever walk again, let alone ski. The notion that Phil would compete in skiing after this injury seemed far-fetched to most people. After extensive surgery that required several screws and a plate to reassemble his ankle, Phil not only returned to skiing, but returned to highly successful competitive skiing. Ultimately, he achieved a goal that was considered unreachable. He won an Olympic silver medal in 1980 and a gold medal in 1984.

Martina Navratilova's tendinitis was so severe that she was contemplating retirement. After non-operative therapy failed to help her, we decided surgery was necessary. During an arthroscopic procedure, we removed tissue that was pulling on the tendon. After successful rehabilitation, she returned to competition and played four more years, winning numerous titles, including two Wimbledon championships.

Chondromalacia sufferers are usually helped with rehabilitation. In some cases, surgery may be necessary. Bruce Smith was considering retirement from professional football in 1991. He had a knee problem with chondromalacia, which was so severe in the patellofemoral joint that he was unable to be competitive. After arthroscopic surgery and extensive rehabilitation, he returned to be a perennial All-Pro and defensive Player of the Year in the NFL.

Those with cartilage defects (a hole in the cartilage created by an injury) can be helped with surgery. Football player Rod Woodson had an injury in 1991 that took away both cartilage and bone from his knee. He had a surgical procedure that we describe as a microfracture; this operation helped regenerate cartilage in the defect created by his injury. After extensive rehabilitation, he returned to his career and was named defensive Player of the Year by the NFL.

A torn ACL does not mean the end of running, tennis or basketball for most patients. At the Steadman-Hawkins Clinic, I have treated numerous professionals in soccer, football, basketball, skiing, and other sports. These athletes have come back to the same or higher levels of performance after treatment and rehabilitation. All of these examples serve as inspiration to the knee pain sufferer.

In ACL surgery, I use the patellar tendon graft as the ligament replacement. This operation is performed only after swelling has gone down and full mobility is achieved. Following surgery, we again try to achieve early full range of motion and decrease the inflammation from surgery. Once mobility is obtained, we start a gradual strengthening program to bring the patient back to full activity.

Knee joint replacement is, or should be, the last resort of

people with severe knee pain. Unfortunately, it is sometimes prematurely recommended to patients.

Choosing a Good Knee Doctor

This book will provide valuable information to those who need the expertise of the best specialists. Graduation from medical school is an important achievement, to be sure. However, the diploma alone does not provide the physician with the knowledge and experience required to treat knee problems. Years of additional training are necessary, *and it is the patient's responsibility* to identify the orthopedists who are the best knee doctors.

The knee is a complicated and invaluable joint deserving the best care available. The extra effort and time spent on identifying an excellent specialist will be the first step in assuring a successful recovery.

Techniques for choosing the best physicians are described in detail in this book. It also provides the reader with the necessary background information on issues that doctors should consider in treatment, such as exercise, diet, treatment modalities, rehabilitation and other factors that are critically important to those seeking a return to physical activity.

An Educated Patient Is a Powerful Patient

Learning how to evaluate the qualifications of various knee doctors is an educational process that this book provides. In addition, it contains details about knees and their problems that will equip the reader to carry on an intelligent discussion with the knee specialist. Ultimately, the doctor will provide the patient with details about his or her knee and its condition.

Based on this, the patient must decide whether or not to choose surgery. A non-operative treatment may also be an option. Armed with the information in this book, an individual can make a wise decision regarding his or her course of treatment. Readers will learn that they have much responsibility in their successful recovery from knee problems. They will learn how to prevent recurrence of injury, and what they can do to maintain good knee function.

J. Richard Steadman, M.D.
Steadman-Hawkins Clinic
Vail, Colorado

INTRODUCTION

About Self-Help

The authors of this book come from different worlds. Dr. John Garrett is an orthopedic surgeon who has spent the majority of his life repairing damaged knees. With a master's in business administration, Bob Reznik specializes in healthcare and the development of centers of excellence, which specialize in caring for patients with certain health problems.

Even with their divergent backgrounds, both share a common belief: The best way to ensure the highest level of quality in healthcare—which means the best possible outcome in terms of function and relief of pain—is to become knowledgeable about your particular problem.

Unlike your parents, who most likely treated the doctor as a god and never asked questions, we encourage you to ask questions freely. That is your right as a patient and a consumer. If you were buying a car, you might spend weeks to educate yourself on the best model for your needs. But when it comes to health, we often blindly follow a single recommendation without really understanding why.

It is important to understand what the doctor is saying. If the doctor is using complicated terms that you don't understand, ask him or her to rephrase in words you will understand. Remember, you are the customer. If your doctor has a problem with an informed patient, beware. You may want to switch. The best doctors understand that a well-informed patient will take responsibility for his or her health. This patient is more likely to stick with the prescribed rehabilitation program.

This book is written because we know that people self-diagnose and medicate themselves—often incorrectly.

The intent of this book is to provide you with information to empower you to make informed choices. Remember: No doctor or nurse can diagnose without a full exam. Neither can you become an orthopedic surgeon and self-diagnose simply by reading a book. There are generalities that are not intended to be applied to your specific condition. To truly discover the cause of your knee problem, you may have to see a knee physician who, by examination and diagnostic tests, will determine the cause of your problem.

Part 1

About Knees

4

Chapter 1

Everything You Need to Know about Knees

If you have knee pain, rest assured you are far from alone. Each year 6 million Americans seek medical help for painful knees. This translates into 2.5 percent of the U.S. population sitting in doctors' offices for relief of knee pain. Even more self-diagnose and treat themselves with pills and home remedies.

The knee is a complex mechanism, which absorbs shock as we jump, and is extremely flexible, permitting change in direction while running at high speeds. It is made of ligaments, which provide support, and muscles for strength. It is a well-lubricated mechanism, which functions reliably unless unduly twisted, bruised, or broken. When this happens problems occur. It is not surprising of all the areas treated by orthopedic surgeons, the knee is the most commonly injured joint, representing 26 percent of orthopedic business, followed by the spine (17 percent) and hip (15 percent).

Often knee pain is the result of an accident, such as a fall or a car crash. Fractures are common. According to the American Academy of Orthopedic Surgeons (AAOS), over a lifetime, each American will suffer two fractures. Many of which will occur at the knee. However, trauma represents a relatively small percentage of knee problems. The vast majority result from repetitive trauma, or wear and tear. In these cases, the cartilage or joint surfaces are slowly damaged over time. One such form of chronic injury is arthritis, which might be thought of as a "rusting" of the knee joint. It causes pain and robs the knee of flexibility. Indeed, half of all knee pain may be tied in some way to arthritis.

Why can't the knees stand up to these demands? Any mechanical device can and will fail if placed under undo strain.

Sometimes knee pain is the result of an accident, such as a fall down stairs or the knee being banged into a dashboard during a car accident. But this is in a relatively small percentage of cases. The vast majority of knee problems develop not from a single accident or fall, but rather over a period of years. In these cases, the knee becomes like a creaky or unstable hinge that doesn't get better, either because components in the knee are weak or unstable, or the lubricating pads and bone surface have been damaged over time.

That's the bad news. The good news is that of all the bum knees that come limping into doctors' offices every year, only 20 percent will need surgery. Of those that don't need surgery, most will get better with time. Anti-inflammatories and specialized exercises that increase range of motion, flexibility, strength, and resistance to future knee strain are usually prescribed. Sometimes knee braces are also used. That's positive news to focus on.

Aside from car accidents, slips, and falls, knees are injured merely from hauling us around all day long. Although we want to stay active, Americans are eating more. The U.S. Government now estimates that 56 percent of Americans are now classified as overweight. This extra weight puts an extra load on aging knees.

Why can't the knee withstand all these extra demands? With undue strain, any mechanical device will fail over time. The knee is a complex hinge designed by Mother Nature. It includes an ingenious mechanism that absorbs shock as we jump from heights, twists when we are running at high speed and change direction, and jacks up heavy loads like a hydraulic lift. Around this hinge are tendons, ligaments, and muscles which provide lateral support and strength.

This wonderful knee mechanism comes with a lifetime supply of hinge lubricant, just so long as the hinge isn't banged, twisted, bruised, or broken. When that happens, serious problems begin.

Arthritis, a form of natural rust, can also cause knee pain. Arthritis is a nasty disease—often inherited and usually associated with aging—which erodes the natural flexibility of a joint. As mentioned, half of knee pain can be tied in some way to arthritis.

Who Can Benefit from This Book

Are you a baby boomer? If so, the statistics for your generation are unique and impressive: There were 78 million babies born between 1946-1964, making it the largest population boom in American history. Additionally, it came at a time of postwar prosperity, when the middle class established home ownership and two-car families.

Through its attitudes and buying behavior this group has reshaped American society. If you're a baby boomer, you know firsthand that you're no longer a kid. If you were born in 1950, you will turn fifty with the turn of the millennium. The raw number of people over sixty years old will jump dramatically from 2010 to 2030 as baby boomers rush headlong into old age. Just like a car hitting 100,000 miles, as the boomers age, the original parts will begin to show signs of wear. Unlike previous generations, baby boomers pose new challenges to the nation's health care system. Not only have baby boomers expanded the midlife percentage of the current total population, they also have a much different attitude about their aches and pains.

Just as most baby boomers feel entitled to an affluent life-style, many feel entitled to an active retirement. Whereas previous generations resigned themselves to the aches and pains of growing older, and lowered their level of activity accordingly, the "Me generation" expects to remain active. They are simply not content to grow old without a fight. That's why marketers are busy creating so many ads aimed at the active senior.

Staying Active As You Age

A new term coined over the last ten years is the "weekend warrior": that middle-aged woman or man who works a desk job during the week, and then on Saturday morning jumps into a full-blown weekend of physical activity. Not surprisingly, by Sunday evening, these warriors are often gobbling Motrin for relief of aches and pains.

Most of us can expect to live longer than our parents. If we make smart decisions about preventing injury and disease, we should be able to stay active into our seventies and eighties, if not longer. Orthopedic surgeons have the task of keeping boomers active. While our original parts may wear out, doctors are discovering new ways to repair or replace them.

Just How Long Can the Original Parts Last?

Just as most people have beliefs about the life span of a car—whether it's 100,000, 200,000, or 300,000 miles—most people have assumptions about what we should expect from our bodies. These assumptions change over time. For instance, in the 1700s, when American society was establishing its roots in the early colonial United States, an "old-timer" was a man or woman in his or her forties. But thanks to advances in health care and diet, the average life span for has increased dramatically. Diseases like polio have been eradicated, and others, such as pneumonia, are no longer fatal. While cancer continues to be the leading cause of death, it can be detected earlier and treated more successfully. Consequently, the average American man will live to seventy-one, and the average American woman can expect to live to seventy-eight.

Have we squeezed the most out of our bodies by living into our seventies? Unlikely. Health experts predict that the number of people living to over one hundred years old will increase dramatically.

So, how long can we realistically expect to live, and how long can we expect our original parts—like our knees—to last? Would you believe to age 120?

Beginning in 1984, the MacArthur Foundation assembled experts from the fields of biology, genetics, and neuroscience to study how humans age and more importantly, to find ways we can live and remain active longer. They released their findings in 1998 in a book entitled *Successful Aging*. The researchers revealed that as recently as the turn of the century, few Americans lived past one hundred years. By 1982, the number of Americans aged one hundred years or older increased to 32,000. By 1997, the number almost doubled. They estimate that at this rate, the number will increase nearly ten times to 600,000 by 2050. The researchers determined, however, that there are realistic limits to the human life span. They found that in almost every species the maximum life span is six times the time required to grow to biological maturity. This formula applies to all beings from fruit flies to humans.

Assuming that it takes humans eighteen to twenty years to reach biological maturity, the researchers calculated a theoretical human life span upwards of 120 years old.

The MacArthur Foundation experts argue that our fate is more closely associated with the choices made over a lifetime. The old person, they explain, *is the cumulative result of the lifestyle chosen over the course of their years.* They maintain that just because your father died of a heart attack does not necessarily give you, the son or daughter, a death sentence at age sixty.

Your Current Choices Will Affect Your Retirement

The experts also note that the picture of the eighty-year-old as a frail and brittle, wheelchair-bound person is a myth. They maintain that Americans can indeed slow the aging process by making choices about fitness—especially as they progress through middle-age in their forties and fifties.

Co-author Bob Reznik remembers as a youngster playing golf with his forty-five-year-old dad. Both father and son carried their golf clubs. They would tee off at dawn, and play until they were losing sight of the ball at dusk. Back then, both routinely played thirty-six, and sometimes fifty-four, holes in a day, walking hilly golf courses, their clubs on their backs.

What is the cumulative result of Dad's lifestyle and choices? Today, he's in his eighties, still playing eighteen holes of golf, shooting a competitive score in the eighties, and still carrying a lightweight carry bag with about eight essential clubs. John's main frustration is that he has to compete with "long-ball hitters" in their fifties because most of his peers are now underground. Following in Dad's footsteps, Bob, now also forty-five, still walks and carries his clubs, even though many of his friends choose to exercise only their right foot as they zoom along the cart path.

Choosing to Stay Active

For middle-aged baby boomers interested in staying active, there are several avenues worth considering. Tennis, an active sport, which has slid from its peak popularity of the late 1970s, deserves a second look. Running, cycling, swimming, and skiing are also good, noncompetitive fitness choices for slowing the aging process for those forty or fifty years old.

Can you remain active into old age? Researchers say it is possible—if you make the proper fitness choices in middle age. They add that there is no reason why original equipment, like your knees, shouldn't last if you make healthy choices. That means being careful about injury.

However, if you've already injured your knee, and pain is preventing you from walking a golf course, playing basketball or skiing, alternatives are available for repair and recovery.

The Knee Is the Crux, or Crutch, of It All

It is difficult to stay active when your knees hurt. They are the linchpin of mobility. When our knees hurt, we are literally stuck. Even getting an aerobic workout for our heart is difficult. Having sore knees can be psychologically devastating. You can feel trapped in a creaky body. However, there is reason for optimism. Many people recover from knee pain. Some even regain peak performance.

For example, pro tennis players give their knees a pounding. Few people are aware that champion Stefan Edberg, widely regarded as one of the best serve and volley artists of tennis, suffered throughout his career from patellar tendinitis, which make it painful to squat. Somehow, he managed to deal with this as he sprinted to the net and lunged for stab volleys.

Likewise, in the final year of her career, Steffi Graf bounced back from knee surgery to win the French Open and make the finals at Wimbledon in 1999 before retiring that year.

How long is the road back from a wounded knee? That can depend on desire to regain top form. Case in point: Pro tennis player Richard Krajicek had knee surgery in November of 1998, and within three months defeated Pete Sampras, the number-one ranked tennis player, in straight sets.

Such success stories provide encouragement. We understand that observing others gives us strength to overcome obstacles. Consequently, in this book, we profile patients who having undergone treatment, successfully recovered, and regained an active life.

How We Live Can Affect Our Knees

Considering how much we depend on our knees, it's surprising how little attention we give them, until they cause us pain. Most people never stretch, even though a common problem associated with excessive sitting is that the hamstrings shorten and cause restricted movement.

Similarly, we load on extra body weight which makes the daily job of carrying us around even more difficult. As we age, we expect the knees to retain the resiliency that they had when we were young. We try to ski the same slopes and moguls at the same speed, and with the same abandon as when we were young.

Around sixty, many knees give out. They just won't carry us anymore. For those who wish to be active, today's surgeons have a last-resort procedure: "total knee replacement." As the term implies, the surgeon replaces the worn-out knee with a man-made joint.

Each year, there are more than 200,000 of these total knee replacement surgeries in the United States. About 65 percent of total knee replacements are done on women, with an average age of 68.7 years old. About 25 percent of all knee replacements are done on middle-aged men and women between forty-five and sixty-four years old.

How This Book Can Help Your Knee Problem

If you are one of the many people with knee pain, this book will provide useful information to help you determine:

1. the cause of pain,
2. if and how it can be treated without surgery, and
3. what to do if nonsurgical treatment doesn't work.

If you need surgery, we'll provide information that will help you locate the best knee surgeons. Orthopedic doctors who treat knees exclusively are often more experienced and proficient than those generalists who treat a variety of orthopedic problems, such as shoulder or spine. Generally speaking, should you go to the older doctor who ostensibly has more years in practice, and hence more experience, or the younger doctor? You may be surprised, but in some cases, the younger doctor may be a better bet.

Younger doctors recognize the need to specialize. The AAOS reports that of those orthopedic surgeons under forty years old, 54 percent have completed a fellowship program— the highest educational level possible—in a certain specialty including hand, spine, knee, or sports medicine. This is compared to only 25 percent of orthopedic surgeons fifty and over. Younger orthopedic surgeons finish a fellowship in which the most advanced knee surgery is performed, working under the watchful eye of a prominent expert. An older, generalist orthopedic surgeon who does knees, ankles, shoulders, and elbows, may not be similarly experienced. Also, generalists may have an annual volume of knee surgeries far less than an orthopedic surgeon who focuses on knee surgery alone. What is the number of knee surgeries per year needed to stay proficient? That's a subject of debate. Some large employers and managed care companies feel that one hundred suggests that a surgeon is proficient and sees a high volume of such cases.

When it comes to surgery, ignorance is not bliss. You need to know what is to be done, and how it will be accomplished. Consequently, we've presented actual photos of two common knee surgeries: replacement of the torn anterior cruciate ligament (torn ACL) and total knee replacement surgery. Once you see these surgeries you will begin to understand the importance of detail, and that surgeons vary in their expertise. We will suggest ways to select the best possible knee surgeon in your area and locate regional Centers of Excellence.

Consider also that just like many other problems, there may be the potential for being too aggressive with treatment. Author and television medical reporter, Dr. Robert Arnot, notes in his book, *The Best Medicine,* that about 6 to 8 percent of knee arthroscopies are done unnecessarily. He adds that of those arthroscopies performed, there are complications in 8 percent of cases.

Ask Questions, Be Informed, and Seek Out the Best Quality Care

Another key difference between the baby boom generation and previous generations, is that baby boomers are the best-informed and educated group of Americans in history. Unlike previous midlifers, this is a generation of skeptics who quiz their doctors, and often seek second opinions. It is a generation that buys books and surfs the Internet to become well-informed on a particular health problem.

In the future, well-informed consumers, like you, will drive quality health care. Doctors will be queried by consumers: "Why is surgery necessary?" Or, "Why can't I become active again?"

Where Does Knee Pain Come From?

Many active people have knee problems. Some are structural. With others, it's a result of inadequate conditioning. Knee pain has impacted the lives of newscaster Walter Cronkite and President Clinton, and has changed the sports careers of tennis greats Steffi Graf and Thomas Muster, and Olympic skier Picabo Street.

Who is at risk? Certainly those who make a living in a career that involves repetitive twisting, stopping, starting, and jumping. Football players are at especially high risk of a sideways blow to the knee while a cleated foot is planted. Basketball players may be injured from jumping. Strains occur from baseball as well as racquetball.

Do knees really wear out with age? Why does a tennis champion like Steffi Graf—who is known for her awesome level of fitness and conditioning—suddenly have her career derailed by a serious knee problem in her twenties, while another tennis great, Jimmy Connors in his mid forties keeps pounding competitors into the court on the senior tour? After all those matches, why didn't his knees wear out? And, why are there healthy middle-aged marathon runners? We'll try to explain this paradox in this book.

Aging baby boomers might also be of higher than normal risk, where poor conditioning matched with overuse, joint strain, and joint degeneration can combine with the natural onset of arthritis.

Women may not play much football, but they have plenty of knee problems. The September-October 1998 issue of the *American Journal of Sports Medicine* reports that women injure their anterior cruciate ligament (ACL) four to eight times more often than men. Why? It's thought that the menstrual cycle and estrogen levels may affect susceptibility to injury.

Differences in pelvic structure between men and women may also be an issue. A woman's pelvis, which is wider, creates a sharper angle between the calf and thigh, increasing pressure on the knee. In addition, a woman's kneecap rides in a shallower groove, making the mechanism less stable.

Another factor discovered by researchers at the University of Michigan is that women don't use their quadriceps and hamstring muscles in the same way as men. Men are equally reliant on the quadriceps and hamstrings, whereas women tend to rely more on their quadriceps during sports activities.

Lastly, high-heel shoes increase the forces on the knee and contribute to osteoarthritis.

While overweight women are most often the ones to need a knee replacement for worn-out knees in their sixties, simple knee *injuries* occur more frequently in men. In fact, knee pain is one of the top ten reasons men see a doctor. Overall, knee pain occurs more in men because they participate more in sports, and they find knee pain stops them in their tracks.

The Four Most Common Knee Problems

While knee pain can occur for a variety of reasons, most knee problems come from four main areas:

1. *Pain from the kneecap.* Those with kneecap pain typically notice an increase in pain when going up or down stairs, when running downhill, or even while sitting.

2. *Torn meniscus.* The bottom of the femur (thigh bone) and the top of the tibia (shin bone) that come together in the knee joint, are covered by cartilage which enables the bones to glide against each other with a minimal amount of friction. But if the knee is twisted, or banged, the cartilage can become damaged or loosened out of its normal position. A common symptom of this type of injury is that the knee may "catch" or grind at a certain point as it moves through its normal range of motion.

3. *Ligament problems.* If you think of the knee as a hinge between the upper leg and lower leg, it is the awesome work of the supporting muscles, ligaments, and tendons to make sure that it is

supported and working properly—often while the leg is twisting, turning and absorbing shock from jumping. There are four key ligaments that can be injured in the knee:

- Anterior cruciate ligament (ACL) is often the victim of noncontact injury, where the knee is twisted while the foot is planted. You may feel a pop, and the whole knee may give way.
- Posterior cruciate ligament (PCL) injuries can be caused by a blow to the knee, or when the knee is forced backward.
- Medial collateral ligament (MCL) can be injured from a blow to the outside area of the knee.
- Lateral collateral ligament (LCL) injury can be caused by a blow to the inside area of the knee.

4. *Tendon problems.* Sometimes the tendons that attach the kneecap (patella) to the shinbone (tibia) can become inflamed.

Treatment of Knee Pain: Where We've Been

When you go to the doctor, keep in mind that the treatment you receive is based on centuries of trial and error. It is interesting to see how far treatment of knee injuries has progressed.

In the 1700s, people often ended up with a barber surgeon who performed surgery on the painful knee. Others endured bloodletting with leeches, under the belief that this would perhaps reduce swelling and relieve pain.

Arthritis sufferers of that time underwent bizarre treatments ranging from sitting in a uranium mine to eating large amounts of cod-liver oil.

The Civil War inflicted some of the most grisly trauma to limbs. Minie ball ammunition often would shatter bone, beyond a physician's ability to repair. Accordingly, a common tool of the battlefield surgeon was the saw—the result being amputation.

The 1900s saw significant advances. Physicians began to subspecialize. Instead of a doctor performing all types of care, from delivering a baby to surgery, doctors began to focus on specific areas of medicine. The field of bone care developed and was dubbed orthopedics.

The last half of the century yielded tremendous change in the treatment of limb problems. Before 1970, it was commonly believed that injured bones and muscles needed stability to heal. Consequently, many leg injuries were immobilized with plaster of paris casts that froze the limb and prevented movement. This also resulted in permanent stiffness of the limb.

Somewhat later, orthopedic surgeons in the field of sports medicine began to innovate new ways to care for leg and arm injury. They discovered that one of the problems associated with immobilization was that the muscles in the limb shrank and became extremely weak. Additionally, it was very painful to begin normal movement again.

Doctors pondered how to foster healing but prevent muscle weakness and stiffness. Medical manufacturers created new surgical implants, which held the injured bone in place while permitting joint movement. These devices shortened the interval required for immobilization and sped recovery. By the 1980s, surgeons working with athletes found that exercise could be started sooner.

Treatment of Knee Pain: Where We Are Now

Over the span of only the last decade, great advances have occurred. In the 1990s, there have been tremendous improvements thanks to sports medicine clinics.

These clinics evolved from having just general orthopedic surgeons to having a new specialization of doctor. In these centers, specialists reengineered injury rehabilitation.

At some centers, clinical outcome is being documented

and tracked to determine how well patients recover. Patients are surveyed when they first visit the doctor to determine how well they perform various activities, such as walking or climbing stairs. After treatment, their ability is again examined to determine the level of improvement.

Treatment of Knee Pain:
Where We Are Going in the Next Century

Beyond the year 2000, surgical manufacturers will research not only new ways to repair joints, but variations of artificial joints, which perform more like our original equipment. Later we will detail advances in synthetic tendons, implant technology, instrumentation systems, and increasingly popular alternative treatments.

We recognize that baby boomers are seeking information on how alternative medicine providers, holistic health remedies, herbs, vitamins, and magnet therapy can play a role in relieving pain.

For example, the *Journal of the American Medical Association* dedicated the November 4, 1998 issue to the subject of alternative medicine. It reported that expenditures in 1990 for alternative medicine was $13.7 billion. Consider that the total cost of hospitalizations that same year was $12.8 billion.

The study also found that the acceptance of alternative medicine is mushrooming. Americans who use alternative care increased from 34 percent, or 60 million, to 42 percent, or 83 million.

But what really makes sense for knee pain? There are a tremendous number of so-called remedies, which do nothing to improve a problem or lower the risk of injury, and are merely a tempting waste of hard-earned money. We will also discuss what application alternative medicine solutions have in the area of knee problems, what's worth a look, and what's not. We will

also look at some of the braces and orthotics currently being pro-
moted in magazines and on the Internet.

Diagnosing Knee Problems

Diagnosing knee problems can be tricky, partly because of the
subjective nature of pain. The main thing to watch for is sudden
swelling and deformity. Preventive techniques will provide you
with significant insurance for protecting your knees. In later
chapters, we'll give you general tips for stretching and exercising, with attention to specific sports. It's important to realize how
far such information can go in preventing injury. One study from
Denmark showed that a group of downhill skiers significantly
lowered their risk for injury after watching an instructional video.

By the same token, being educated about knee pain, diagnosis and treatment options can ensure that you receive the
best care whether it be home remedies, conventional, or
alternative forms of medicine.

There is much to keep in mind as you strive to become
pain-free, namely that almost all cases of knee pain can be rem-
edied with today's treatments. Knee pain sufferers have found
relief in everything from apitherapy, which is the medicinal application of bee products, to state of the art procedures, including computer-assisted knee replacement surgery.

You should also be aware of little-known facts, like how
having surgery too soon can set your knees back, and that where
you live can determine the treatment you receive. For example,
some cities have a higher incidence of surgery than others. A
few even have a surgical rate that is higher than what is
recommended by the National Institutes of Health.

Any sport can challenge your knees and result in an injury, but the June 1997 Harvard Health Letter identifies the three
sports which pose the greatest threat: tennis, skiing, and basketball. Football and wrestling are sports that yield the highest

number of injuries, but these are not always knee-related. Basically, activities which involve sudden twisting movements are the ones which lead to ligament and cartilage damage. We'll give you some suggestions on how to lessen your risk.

The structure of the knee is what makes it so precarious. The mechanics of the knee are so complex that there are twenty-five to thirty-five types of knee injuries. Just because the knee is prone to injury, however, doesn't necessarily mean it's weak. Amazingly, the knee supports the weight of the entire body.

We'll take a closer look at the structure of the knee, and specific types of injuries especially, in Chapter 2, where you will get a course in knee anatomy.

Chapter 2

Anatomy Lesson

To understand why your knees hurt, you must first get an understanding of how they work. To do that, you need to know a little bit about anatomy.

Healthy knees do their job so well that most of us are oblivious to their complex inner workings. The very structures that allow us to walk, run, jump, and pivot don't command our attention until something goes wrong. In spite of all they do, the bones, ligaments, tendons, and muscles in the knee joint have a thankless job. Some of us are just plain insensitive when it comes to our knees. We expect a lot and give nothing in return. If you're not careful, the misunderstood knee will one day make you sit up or, in some cases, lay down and take notice.

How does the knee accomplish its task? The knee is designed for two principle motions: flexion and extension. As an added benefit, the knee even allows a limited range of rotation. The key word here is "limited." Many knee injuries occur when we push our knee's rotational ability beyond its limits.

What Kind of Joint Is This Anyway?

A joint is the collective term for an assembly of bones and connective tissue structures. Joints are classified by function, whether it's supporting the weight of the body or providing mobility. There are three types of joints: fibrous, cartilaginous, and synovial.

We want to focus on the knees, so we'll stick to the synovial joints, which are representative of the majority of joints in the body, including the knees. The term *synovial* means that the entire joint is encased within a capsule, which acts as a protective sleeve for the complex network of bones, muscles, ligaments, tendons, and cartilage. The lining of this capsule is called the synovium. It secretes a fluid that lubricates the joint.

Synovial joints are known for movement, but not all synovial joints provide motion to the same degree. Your hips, ankles, shoulders, and wrists are also synovial joints. And of all joints, the knee is the most flexible and the most vulnerable to injury.

Bone Up on Your Knee Knowledge

The knee joint is comprised of four bones. The largest of these is the femur, or thigh bone. Also found in the knee is the tibia, sometimes called the shin bone. Alongside the tibia, on the outside of the leg, is the fibula.

The fourth bone found in the knee is the patella or kneecap. It's cradled within the patellar tendon, and lies directly in front of the femur. This patella assists in knee extension, increasing leverage by lifting the quadriceps and patellar tendons away from the joint.

The lower end of the femur is rounded into two knob-shaped masses known as condyles. These move against the upper end of the tibia, which is flat. Both the lower end of the femur and upper end of the tibia are covered with articular

General image of the knee and leg

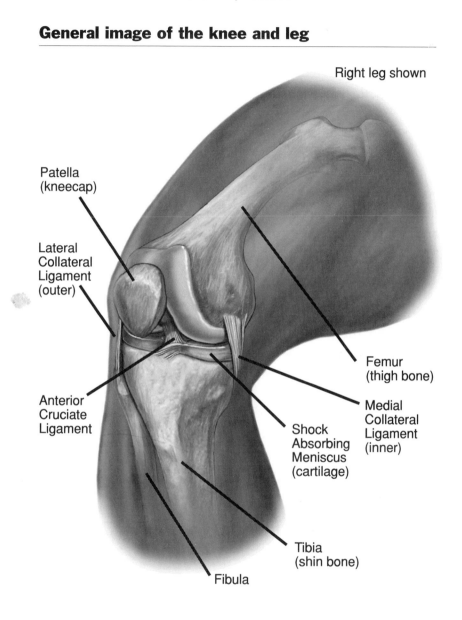

Right leg shown

Patella
(kneecap)

Lateral
Collateral
Ligament
(outer)

Anterior
Cruciate
Ligament

Femur
(thigh bone)

Medial
Collateral
Ligament
(inner)

Shock
Absorbing
Meniscus
(cartilage)

Tibia
(shin bone)

Fibula

cartilage, a smooth rubbery material, which allows one surface to glide one upon the other with minimal friction. Sandwiched between the two joints are two distinct masses of fibrocartilaginous material called menisci, which acts as an additional cushion for the joint.

In addition to the meniscus, there is articular cartilage covering the ends of the femur, the top of the tibia, and the back of the patella. Articular cartilage is found throughout the body anywhere two bones meet and glide against each other. The point of meeting and movement for bones is described as the point of articulation, hence the name "articular cartilage."

Articular Cartilage

As you visualize the bones in the knee joint, consider that if the femur were to move against the tibia, especially under the weight of our bodies, the friction would erode the joint surfaces.

Thankfully, wear is reduced by the articular cartilage on the femur and tibia. The articular cartilage covering the surface of these two bones is about 1/4-inch thick and appears white and shiny and actually has a rubbery feel to it, almost like the chrome on a trailer hitch. The articular cartilage enables the femur and tibia to glide against one another with minimal resistance.

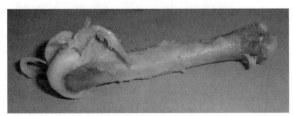

A quick way to learn about cartilage is to take a chicken or turkey leg, and examine the white shiny coating of cartilage at the joint surface. Feel how smooth it is, then take a knife and scrape at the surface. Then feel how the surface has become rough.

Meet the Meniscus

As the largest of joints, and the one bearing the heaviest burden, our knees are fortified with an extra layer of cartilage just between the femur and tibia. The menisci protect the articular cartilage by spreading out the forces placed on the joint surfaces during movement. To imagine how valuable this function is,

Focus on the meniscus and articular cartilage

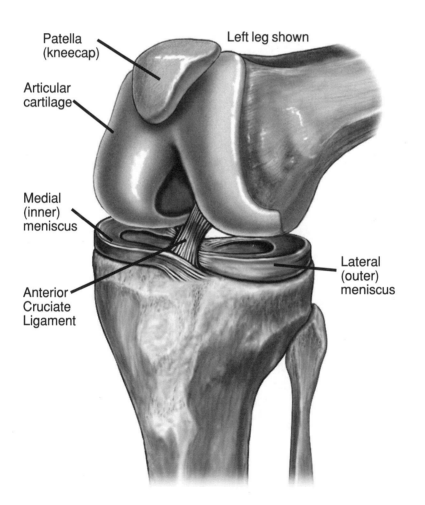

Patella
(kneecap)

Left leg shown

Articular
cartilage

Medial
(inner)
meniscus

Anterior
Cruciate
Ligament

Lateral
(outer)
meniscus

A healthy meniscus (top), and torn meniscus (bottom)

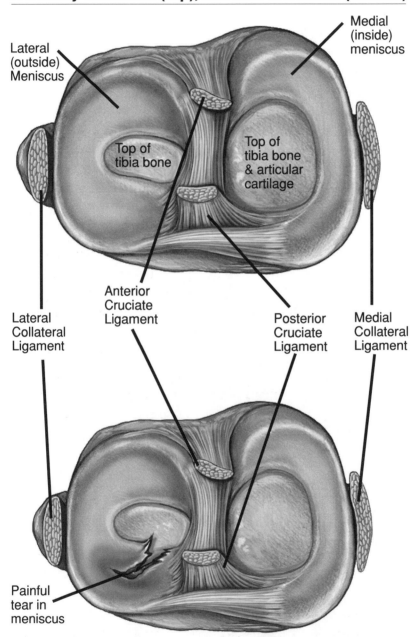

Medial (inside) meniscus

Lateral (outside) Meniscus

Top of tibia bone

Top of tibia bone & articular cartilage

Anterior Cruciate Ligament

Lateral Collateral Ligament

Posterior Cruciate Ligament

Medial Collateral Ligament

Painful tear in meniscus

consider that forces on the knee range from about twice our body weight during normal walking, to more than four times our body weight during running activities.

The meniscus also plays a role in shock absorption. Considering the meniscal layer is only about one-fourth of an inch thick, this padding does a remarkable job of softening impact and vibration when our feet hit the ground walking, running, and jumping. Knees with the menisci in top form have a shock absorption capacity that is 20 percent higher than knees in which the menisci have been removed (*Surgery of the Knee, Vol 1. pg. 25*). This underscores the importance of injury prevention when it comes to the knee. Once you damage the shock absorber, you are that much more susceptible to arthritis.

Menisci also aid the knees in maintaining stability. If you placed a ball on a flat surface, you'd have a pretty good idea of what the knee would be like without the meniscus. Except for the ligaments, there would be nothing to keep the femur from rolling right off the tibia. When we are young, menisci are tough but can tear as a result of a sports injury. As we reach our fifth decade of life, menisci can become fragile and often tear with just a slight twist. During arthroscopic surgery of the knee, a knee surgeon will attempt to clean up and remove the torn part of the meniscus, while at the same time trying to preserve as much of it as possible.

What Are "Ligaments"?

Ligaments interconnect the bones of the knee. They are made up of tough collagen fibers, which themselves are relatively inflexible. However, they are arranged with a crimp design that straightens when force is applied and permits the ligaments to endure large internal stresses during normal joint motion. Ligaments are attached to bone in such a manner that there is progressive increase in stiffness as they blend into bone.

The four key ligaments: ACL, PCL, MCL, LCL

(Right leg viewed from the front)

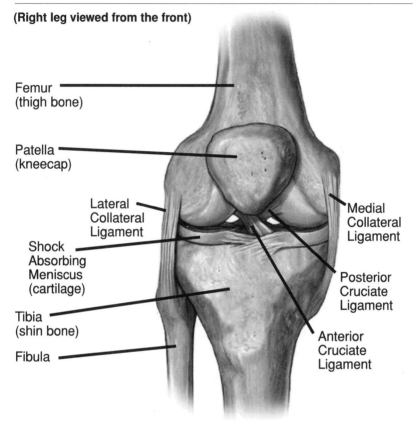

Femur
(thigh bone)

Patella
(kneecap)

Lateral
Collateral
Ligament

Shock
Absorbing
Meniscus
(cartilage)

Tibia
(shin bone)

Fibula

Medial
Collateral
Ligament

Posterior
Cruciate
Ligament

Anterior
Cruciate
Ligament

The way that ligaments become part of a bone is also important to their function. Ligamentous tissue and bone meet together in a graduation of fibrocartilage and mineralized fibrocartilage, which provides the increasing stiffness as ligament blends into bone.

The four major ligaments of the knee are:

     1. the anterior cruciate ligament,
     2. the posterior cruciate ligament,
     3. the medial collateral ligament, and
     4. the lateral collateral ligament.

The stability of the knee is largely due to their combined efforts. They are the structures that ultimately hold the tibia and femur together, while permitting motion.

The anterior cruciate ligament (ACL) is deep within the knee. It crisscrosses the posterior cruciate ligament (PCL) and keeps the tibia from sliding too far forward in relation to the femur. The PCL does the opposite. It prevents the tibia from sliding excessively backwards. The PCL is further supported by two minor ligaments: the ligaments of Humphry and Wrisberg.

Muscles related to the knee

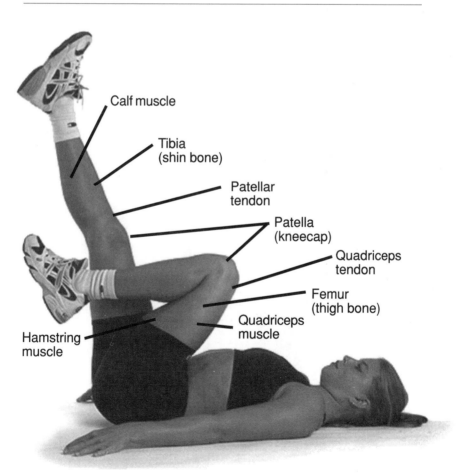

Calf muscle

Tibia
(shin bone)

Patellar
tendon

Patella
(kneecap)

Quadriceps
tendon

Femur
(thigh bone)

Quadriceps
muscle

Hamstring
muscle

The ligaments that provide sidewise stability to the knee are the medial collateral ligament (MCL) and lateral collateral ligament (LCL). These ligaments limit side-to-side motion.

Tendons, Muscles, Nerves, Blood Vessels in the Knee

Tendons are cords of strong, fibrous tissue, which connect muscle to bone. Muscle power is transferred across tendons to bones. The primary muscle groups associated with the knee are the quadriceps and hamstring muscles. These muscles are at work when the knee is extended, flexed, or rotated.

Muscles related to the knee joint

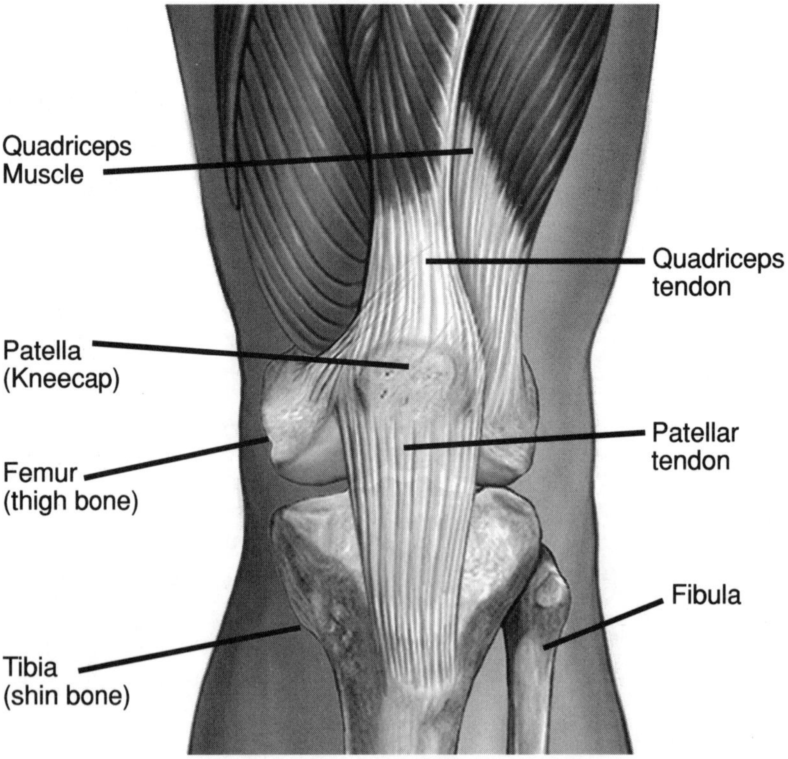

Quadriceps Muscle

Quadriceps tendon

Patella (Kneecap)

Patellar tendon

Femur (thigh bone)

Fibula

Tibia (shin bone)

The easiest way to understand how the muscles in the leg operate is to imagine two large rubber bands, one that runs down the front, and another that runs down the back. The front rubber band pulls the leg straight, or extends it. The rear rubber band causes the leg to do the reverse, or flexes it.

The quadriceps mechanism is the strongest muscle in the leg, allowing us to walk and run. The quadriceps mechanism includes:

1. quadriceps muscle,
2. quadriceps tendon above the patella,
3. patella, and
4. patellar tendon.

The quadriceps tendon connects the quadriceps muscle to the patella, while the patellar tendon connects the patella to the tibia. The hamstring muscles at the back of the thigh, as well as the calf muscles, enable the knee to flex.

Working together, the muscles, tendons, and ligaments of the knee work fluidly. Turn to any sports channel on a Sunday afternoon and pay attention to the slow motion videos of a wide receiver running a complex pass route, jumping through the air to snatch a football, and then changing directions and accelerating into the end zone. Or watch a skier charge through a slalom course, knees pumping as they work the edges of their skis through the gates.

That's when everything is working perfectly. Things change after a wide receiver takes a blow to the side of the knee, or when that downhill skier catches an edge and tumbles.

Now that you have an understanding of the gears and moving parts that make up the knee joint, we start to understand what can go wrong.

Part 2

Knee Pain and Its Causes

Chapter 3

What Causes Knee Pain?

Pain is the principal reason we visit the doctor. Pain is our natural, biological alarm, which warns us that something is wrong and often is a signal to stop before permanent damage occurs.

According to *U.S. News & World Report*, 34 million Americans suffer from chronic pain which eventually takes its toll on quality of life, personal income, and productivity. Americans spend more than $40 billion for relief from body aches. Of those with arthritis, one out of three has to limit daily activities.

When you consider that in the United States one of every four sick days taken—50 million work days total—is because of pain, it becomes clear that it is a significant problem.

An aspect of pain that is troubling to doctors, is that it is subjective. People are surprised to learn that there is no diagnostic test that will confirm the presence of pain or measure its severity. With all of medicine's advances, we still are left to measure pain based on a person's subjective perception of it. Doctors, for example, use pain scales that ask a patient how bad their pain is on a one to ten scale, with ten being excruciating.

To understand pain better, we need to define the common terms "acute" and "chronic" pain, as well as discuss pain which results from strains, sprains, and tears.

Acute and Chronic

Acute pain is sudden and immediately follows injury. It is often severe and stabbing in contrast to the dull sensation of chronic pain. Meniscal and ligament tears and fractures often produce acute pain. It is important to realize that acute pain may subside or resolve completely with time, but quite often it may evolve into chronic pain.

On the other hand, chronic discomfort is persistent pain, or pain that surfaces intermittently over the course of time. Chronic discomfort often is associated with degenerative problems. Arthritis, chondromalacia, patella, bursitis, patellar tendinitis, and iliotibial band syndrome are just a few knee problems that fall under its umbrella.

Strains, Sprains, and Tears

Strains are common and occur when a muscle is overworked or overstretched. When you suddenly dive into a new activity or exercise program, you often strain a muscle or tendon by overworking it. A strained muscle is what we sometimes call a "pulled" muscle. A strain is characterized by a sharp pain or "stitch" at the time of injury. The area becomes sore and stiff within a few hours or moments of straining. Pain accompanies further movement but often subsides within days.

Strains often occur when, after months of inactivity, we throw ourselves into a new exercise routine. If you are out of shape and haven't carefully stretched your muscles, think twice before zealously jumping on the treadmill and powering it up to a high-speed performance level. When the machine starts racing, your legs might race right out from under you, and in that case, you'll be lucky if a strain is the only injury suffered.

Sprains are more serious than strains. A sprain occurs when a *ligament* is overstretched or partially torn. Since ligaments hold bones together, their close proximity to the bone may lead to the suspicion of a fracture. The signs of a sprain include joint pain, which increases with movement, tenderness to the touch, and rapid swelling. These may be associated with black and blue discoloration. Sprains in the knee involve partial tears to the ACL, PCL, MCL, and LCL.

The location of the injury should clarify any confusion over whether it's a sprain or strain. Strains occur in the muscles of the neck, back, thighs, and calves. Sprains are found around joints—knees, ankles, or wrists.

Tears are more severe than strains or sprains. When muscles, ligaments, or tendons are torn they are actually disrupted. The torn ends grossly disrupt the continuity of their structure.

What Is Inflammation?

The word "inflammation" literally means to "set on fire." Its characteristics are swelling, reddening, pain, and heat. Inflammation is a defensive reaction to injury. There are hundreds of inflammatory processes, as indicated by the "-itis" suffix. Tendinitis, bursitis, and arthritis are conditions which bring about inflammation in the knee.

What's good about inflammation? Each characteristic of inflammation provides a clue. The reddened appearance of inflamed tissue is a result of an increased blood supply. This carries white blood cells to the affected tissues. These are the agents which release enzymes to aid in healing or destroy germs.

This extra concentration of blood cells and fluid causes the area to swell, while increased local metabolism increases warmth. Pain occurs as a result of these processes and often prompts one to seek care. Inflammation may be present both in acute or chronic knee problems.

Pain from Meniscus Tears

Meniscal tears can occur at any age. In the younger age group, they are usually sports-related and result from violent trauma. Contact sports like football account for a large number of tears. The type of movement that most often causes meniscal injury is one in which the foot is firmly planted on the ground while the knee is twisted. Shoes with cleats often contribute to this type of injury by anchoring the lower leg into the ground and preventing it from moving with the knee.

Along with other sports, which call for cutting, pivoting, or decelerating, basketball and tennis can also lead to meniscal tears. Traumatic meniscal injuries may also be accompanied by the tearing of a ligament, such as the anterior cruciate ligament.

For those forty and older, meniscal tears are less likely to be due to sports injury. With age the meniscus weakens and

Pain from a torn meniscus

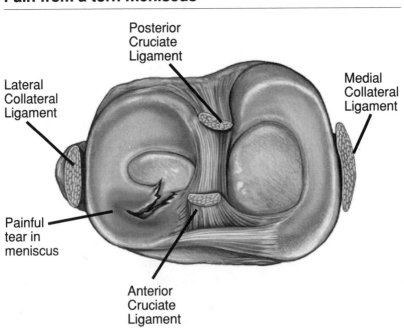

Posterior Cruciate Ligament

Lateral Collateral Ligament

Medial Collateral Ligament

Painful tear in meniscus

Anterior Cruciate Ligament

becomes more fragile. Individuals in this age group can tear a meniscus by performing simple activities, such as squatting.

Meniscal tears come in a variety of sizes and shapes. Often torn fragments lodge between the tibia and femur causing mechanical obstruction and pain. When this happens, the knee is said to "lock up" which means that the patient is unable to extend the knee fully outward. Fluid accumulates as the result of an inflammatory process, and walking becomes difficult.

Menisci lack blood supply except at their outer rim. Once torn, they heal poorly, if at all, and function is lost. Symptoms often vary in intensity depending upon the level of one's activity.

Chondromalacia

"Chondro" indicates *cartilage*, while "malacia" means *softening*. Consequently, chondromalacia together means softening of the cartilage.

But chondromalacia really refers specifically to softening of the under surface of the patella, or kneecap. It is a degenerative condition which occurs as the result of chronic wear of the kneecap against the femur. The articular cartilage gradually softens and then frays.

At other times, a traumatic blow around the knee is the cause of chondromalacia. Symptoms of chondromalacia include pain in front of the knee, especially when walking up and downhill, stiffness after prolonged sitting, and a grinding or clicking sensation as the knee is flexed and extended.

Symptoms typically vary according to the level of activity and may limit one's participation in sports. As problems progress, patients may also lose speed and strength, and notice swelling. The condition is increasingly common in middle age. For reasons unknown, it occurs most in women, and may begin as early as the teenage years.

It has even been suggested that some people may be

predisposed to chondromalacia. Women suffer most from this condition possibly due to muscle weakness in the extension mechanism and anatomical factors, which cause the kneecap to slip out of alignment. Symptoms may be especially severe with repetitive activities like running or aerobics, although cyclists are not immune to the problem.

Ligament Problems

Every year there are more than 50,000 hospital admissions for ligament repair. The number of these injuries grows each year. What is causing the increase?

The steady increase in ACL injuries is due partly to the increasing number of Americans participating in sports; thanks to government legislation, this includes women. In 1972, Title IX mandated equal educational rights in sports for women. Accordingly, they have moved into sports in droves, bringing with them a higher incidence of anterior cruciate ligament injury per sports event. According to a 1998 *San Francisco Examiner* report, during the 1989-1990 intercollegiate basketball season, women injured their ACL 7.8 times more than men.

Certain ligaments are especially vulnerable. The ACL and MCL are the most commonly torn. Frequent causes of ligament injuries include twisting or changing direction rapidly, slowing down when running, and landing from a jump. Specific athletes at risk are those who ski, play basketball, soccer, or football.

Why are ligaments so easily damaged? Consider the average size of the ACL or PCL. They're smaller than you might think. The ACL is about one centimeter wide and has a range of eight to thirteen millimeters wide, while the PCL is thirteen to sixteen millimeters. Both of these ligaments are only about four centimeters in length.

The Torn ACL Ligament

The sound of an ACL as it tears is distinctive, and the the feeling unforgettable. Here's what happens.

The anterior cruciate ligament tightens as the knee is twisted. But when the knee is forced past the normal straightened position, or when the tibia is twisted excessively outward on the femur, or frequently when the knee is struck from the side, the ACL may be stretched beyond its breaking point.

Those nearby will notice a distinctive popping sound, and the afflicted individual will experience a sudden burst of pain and instability. Often the knee buckles, causing a fall to the floor. Swelling appears promptly.

Swelling and pain may subside, but after returning to sports, there will be a sense of instability with any twisting maneuver. While not commonly the case, bleeding may occur in the knee. Because the knee is now rendered unstable, repeated injury can now damage the menisci or articular cartilage and ultimately lead to arthritis.

Other Ligament Tears

Of all the ligaments, the one least likely to be injured is the posterior cruciate. It is commonly injured by a direct blow to the front of the shin, with the knee flexed. This may occur when a football player falls against the ground with a flexed knee or in a car accident, in which the shin is driven into the dashboard while the knee is flexed.

Injuries to the medial or lateral collateral ligaments are often suffered when the knee is struck from the outside or inside or can be a subsequent result of twisting injuries, when first the anterior cruciate ligament and then a collateral ligament ruptures.

A blow to the outside of the knee can occur in contact sports like football. With slighter injuries, the individual may simply feel pain but be able to continue playing until he or she notices stiffness. Unlike anterior cruciate injuries, injuries solely to a collateral ligament do not produce swelling.

In extreme cases of trauma, as may occur in a car accident, multiple ligaments may rupture. The knee may in fact completely dislocate, causing damage to three or more ligaments.

Unlike menisci, ligaments have an ample blood supply. Of the two cruciate ligaments, the anterior cruciate is most often injured. When the ligament is injured, both the structural integrity of the ligament and its blood supply are lost. The residual ligamentous mass shrivels, leaving the knee unstable. The amount of instability varies according to the inherent tightness of the knee and other associated ligament injuries. Instability is often an obstacle to patients who wish to remain active, and ligament reconstruction is often necessary.

The easiest way to injure your posterior cruciate ligament is to receive a direct blow to the front of the knee, which forces it to cave backward. Again, contact sports may lead to PCL injury, as do auto accidents in which the knee is slammed into the dashboard. Isolated tears usually heal without catastrophic instability. Surgery is less frequently required.

The MCL and LCL suffer injury when the knee is pushed too far sideways. The MCL is most often injured during a blow to the outer side of the knee, as in football or hockey. The victim of this painful tear may feel the knee "pop" or collapse sideways. Compared to the MCL, injuries to the LCL occur rarely. Injuries isolated to a collateral ligament rarely require surgery.

The average time it takes to heal a ligament sprain depends on the severity of the injury and level of activity. Isolated medial collateral ligament tears may heal in four to six weeks. Partial tears of the ACL, infrequent as they are, do not regain maximum strength for four to six months.

Tendon Trouble

There are four primary problems related to tendons in the knee. The first of these is tendinitis. Tendinitis refers to inflammation, which results from microscopic tears within the tendon fabric. Although the overall integrity of the tendon is maintained, pain may become disabling. Tendinitis is common in the quadriceps and patella tendons. The disorder is often attributed to overuse.

Dancers and runners are frequently afflicted, especially when training excessively. Similarly, those involved in jumping sports, specifically basketball, broad jump, and the long jump are at risk. The problem is so common within these sports that it has gained the label "jumper's knee." Such pain can be annoying and may limit sporting activities, but is usually not catastrophic. Treatment typically involves rest, stretching, and anti-inflammatory medication.

Tendinitis may also be the result of a tendon chafing upon the underlying bony structures, such as when the iliotibial band rubs upon the underlying femur as the knee is flexed and extended. Although the iliotibial band begins at the hip, it does not form a distinct band until it reaches the knee. Each time the knee flexes and extends, this band rubs, albeit gently, against the outer aspect of the femur.

In long distance running, repetitive rubbing of the band against the femur, which may occur thousands of times in relatively quick succession, results in friction, inflammation, and finally pain. It is similar to the way a shoe may rub against a foot, causing a blister. No swelling occurs, but pain can limit running and even cause a limp. Permanent damage does not occur, but because of the need for rest, runners often are frustrated in their attempts to maintain a training program. Anti-inflammatory medication may be of value in reducing pain, but stretching has little if any benefit.

Severe injury can actually tear a tendon. This typically involves either the patellar or quadriceps tendon. When it occurs, the result is catastrophic. The connection between the quadriceps muscle and extensor mechanism is disrupted and contractions of the quadriceps muscle no longer produce extension of the knee.

The injury often occurs as a result of a fall upon a flexed knee. Younger people are more at risk of tearing a patellar tendon; those of advanced age are more susceptible to tears of the quadriceps tendon. President Clinton is a good example of the latter. Once tendon rupture occurs, disability is severe. Normal activities including walking, running, climbing and descending stairs are severely affected and surgery is indicated.

Arthritis

Arthritis literally means "fire in the joints." People who suffer from the disease can attest to the accuracy of this description. Statistics from the Arthritis Foundation estimate that one in seven Americans is affected. Many are elderly, but arthritis is not a disease which discriminates according to age. It affects every strata of the population, young and old, women more so than men.

Osteoarthritis

Osteoarthritis is the most common form of arthritis and makes a particularly strong showing in the middle aged. The term osteoarthritis is synonymous with "wear and tear" arthritis, or degenerative joint disease. The terms refers to the actual wear and erosion of the articular cartilage, which continues until finally no cartilage remains and bone rubs against bone.

Symptoms include pain, stiffness, and swelling. At first they may be intermittent, but as deterioration progresses, they occur with greater regularity and intensity. When the entire thickness of the articular cartilage has worn away and bone rubs harshly against bone, pain increases dramatically and may be incapacitating.

The tendency to develop osteoarthritis is often inherited. Other factors include injury or repetitive stress from excessive use. Those who are bowlegged or have knock-knees are at increased risk. The last, but perhaps the most common factor is excess body weight.

Pain from degenerative arthritis

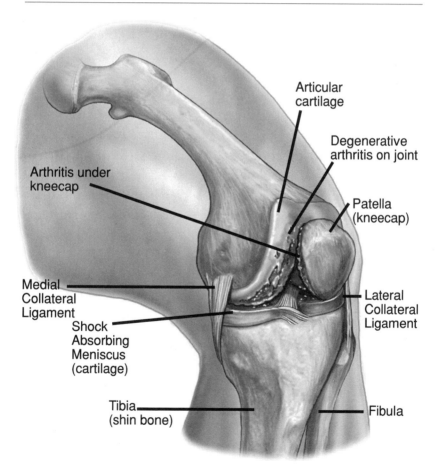

Rheumatoid Arthritis

Rheumatoid arthritis is a second form of arthritis. Instead of a process of wear and tear, it begins with inflammation, which eventually leads to destruction of one or many joints. Its cause is unknown. It affects all age groups, but most often attacks women in middle age. It may attack a single joint, but more commonly simultaneously attacks many joints within the body.

The disease manifests itself in many ways. In some cases the symptoms involve one or two joints, are transient, and vanish without causing permanent damage. More commonly, many joints are affected, rapid deterioration occurs, and joints become grossly deformed. Both large and small joints may be damaged. The knee is often affected along with other large joints such as the hips.

Crystalline Arthritis

The third category of arthritis is "crystalline" arthritis. Two common types are gout and chondrocalcinosis. Gout is a disorder of the body's metabolism where small crystals of sodium urate are deposited within the knee joint. These crystals cause inflammation in the same manner that a small grain of sand may cause inflammation in the eye with resultant tearing.

With chondrocalcinosis the process is similar, but calcium pyrophosphate crystals rather than urate crystals cause the problem. These diseases are characterized by attacks of pain, redness, and swelling of the affected joint. They are common in men over the age of thirty. Women are at low risk until after menopause. These forms of arthritis, although painful during acute episodes, are typically managable.

A Crack or Out of Whack?

The term "fracture" refers to a break in the bony structures. The simplest cases are represented by a crack. In more severe cases, the bony fragments break apart, losing their normal relation point with one another. Fractures are commonly the result of sudden severe injury, such as a fall or vehicular accident. Sometimes they are small, only a small chip breaking loose. At other times, large portions of the joint surface are broken, and the overall structure radically altered. Pain and swelling occur and discoloration may eventually appear. In extreme cases actual deformity of the knee joint or limb may result.

A second type of fracture occurs with repetitive stress. This type of fracture is called a "stress" fracture and is common around the knee. Long distance running or repetitive jumping can result in stress fractures. Often these fractures go undiagnosed because their signs are not overt. Pain is common, but swelling or deformity rarely appear. Routine X-rays may fail to disclose the injury, which is only revealed on a bone scan or MRI.

The older we get, the more thin and fragile the bones become. For women, the possibility of breaking a bone increases with age because of osteoporosis. Women become at increased risk especially after menopause because of diminished estrogen, which normally stimulates bone growth. Although the most common fractures occur around the spine, hip, and wrist, fractures of the knee are not unusual. This includes fractures of the tibia plateau and patella, both of which may be quite disabling.

According to the 1995 records of the National Center for Health Statistics there were 23,000 fractures of the femur among forty-five to sixty-four-year-old men and women.

This age group had the second highest incidence of breaks after the sixty-five and older population. They also ran a close second to the eighteen to forty-four group in fractures of the tibia and fibula. Kneecap fractures weren't common at any age, but that doesn't mean they didn't happen. Four thousand boomers fractured their kneecaps in 1995. If you broke a bone as a kid or teen, don't think the odds are against you breaking another one in this lifetime. The AAOS says that through the course of a lifetime, each one of us will, on average, suffer two fractures.

Fractures in the knee area

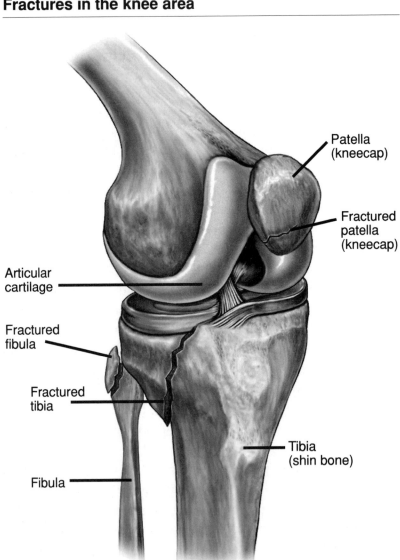

Patella (kneecap)

Fractured patella (kneecap)

Articular cartilage

Fractured fibula

Fractured tibia

Tibia (shin bone)

Fibula

Dislocation

Sometimes bones don't break. Rather, trauma pushes one bone out of alignment with its neighbors. When this happens, a "dislocation" has occurred. A sidewise blow can knock the kneecap out of place. Anatomic differences make some individuals more prone to this type of injury. If the patellar groove in the femur is shallow and ligaments are lax, as is the case with some women, the kneecap can be displaced easily.

Knee Problems That Affect Kids

Knee problems don't just affect the middle-aged. Kids can suffer from their own set of knee problems.

Children are not young adults, nor are they meant to be. Children have inherent weaknesses within their skeleton, which make them prone to a specific set of orthopedic problems. Typically the time of greatest involvement in sports, childhood can bring exposure to knee trauma.

The injuries suffered, however, differ greatly from those seen in adults. For that reason, a parent should take an injured child or teenager to a pediatric orthopedic surgeon, preferably one who specializes in sports medicine. The following categories cover issues that should be considered when an adolescent or teenager is injured.

Knee Fractures in Kids

Many teenagers are still actively growing. The growth plates around the knee, which are on the lower end of the femur and upper end of the tibia, remain open almost until overall height is attained. That is age thirteen to fourteen for girls and fifteen to eighteen for boys.

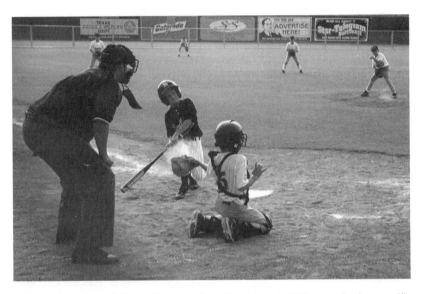

"Mom, my knee hurts." Knee problems aren't just for old people. Kids can suffer from specific tendon problems that affect the young. Knees also take a fair amount of bumps, bruises, and whacks while growing up. Any mom will testify that boys wear out the knees of their pants faster than any other piece of clothing.

Until growth plates close, a twist or a blow to a knee that might tear the anterior cruciate ligament in an adult, often results in fracture in the adolescent knee. The injury is the same, and the pain and swelling identical, but the treatment is quite different.

Unless properly treated, growth plate fracture can result either in cessation of growth in the limb, resulting in a shorter leg, or produce unequal maturation across the width of the growth plate, resulting in bowed leg or knock-knee deformity.

Dislocated Patella in Children

Many children, especially girls, exhibit what is medically termed "hyperlaxity." In common terms, this is known as being "double-jointed." Such individuals can easily do backbends or bend forward at the waist to touch their elbows to the ground.

Often, this excessive play in the joints results in dislocation. This is especially true of the patella. In addition, many of these same individuals have knock-knee deformity and a shallow groove for the patella to ride within. A twisting injury, similar to what might tear an anterior cruciate ligament in an adult, instead causes the patella to dislocate to the outside of the knee. Extreme pain is experienced and the child often ends up in the emergency room having the kneecap put back into proper position.

On other occasions, the patella spontaneously relocates itself or only partially dislocates (subluxes), making a definitive diagnosis somewhat more difficult. Initial dislocations are often treated with immobilization and physical therapy. Recurrent dislocations can lead to damage of the joint surfaces and arthritis. They often require surgery.

Osgood-Schlatter's Disease

Adults who participate in running and jumping sports are prone to patellar tendinitis: "jumper's knee." But youngsters with open growth plates who perform the same activities can suffer from Osgood-Schlatter's disease instead. This is a tendon problem that specifically affects the young, usually during adolescence. Osgood-Schlatter's disease is named after the American and German surgeons who first described the disorder.

The problem arises during adolescent growth spurts. Tension in the patellar tendon where it connects to the growth plate on the upper tibia causes small cracks within the growth plate. Small portions of the growth plate are slowly pulled upwards and away, but not far from their point of origin.

Although overall function of the extensor mechanism remains intact, adolescents experience pain when running and jumping. Tenderness is felt at the site, where swelling and an obvious protuberance appears in front of the knee. Pain may be severe and prevent participation in sports. Symptoms typically abate with rest, but may occur intermittently until growth ceases. Only in a few cases do symptoms persist into adulthood and remain so troublesome that surgery is required.

Pain from damage to articular cartilage

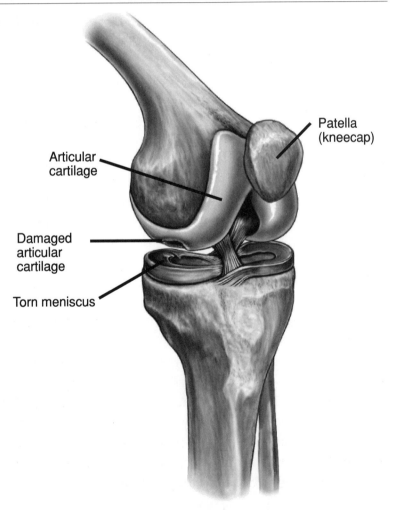

Patella (kneecap)

Articular cartilage

Damaged articular cartilage

Torn meniscus

Anterior Knee Joint Pain/Chondromalacia

Many middle-aged people suffer from chondromalacia. Its symptoms include anterior knee joint pain, a sensation of grinding or popping, and tendon stiffness and swelling. When a physician peers inside the knee with an arthroscope, often there will be clear evidence of wear and tear on the inside of the knee. Years of sports and stress have taken their toll.

Not so with most adolescent knees. Excessive sports or other play activity may cause similar pain, but it does so without the structural damage noted in adults. It is pain that occurs in an otherwise healthy knee. Thus the label, "anterior knee joint pain" rather than chondromalacia. The cause is often the same. The culprit is usually excessive activity, often related to running sports. Track and cross-country can be common causes.

Pain is invariably noted at the front of the knee or beneath the kneecap, but unlike adults, children rarely note the grinding sensation behind the knee that a grown person may complain about. Physical evidence of damage may be absent on a physical exam, and X-rays can appear normal.

As with adults, treatment consists of rest and anti-inflammatory medication. Strengthening exercises can be helpful.

Benign Bone Tumor/Osteochondroma

Occasionally, adolescent knee pain is the result of the presence of a tumor, often entirely benign. One such tumor is an osteochondroma, which is often found on the femur or tibia in proximity of the knee joint. On X-rays, these have the appearance of a bony hook and often can be felt beneath the skin as a hard mass. The overlying muscle often rubs over the tumor causing pain or even a snapping sensation as the knee is flexed and extended. These tumors are mostly benign and therefore harmless, but frequently must be removed because of pain.

Osteochondritis Dissecans

Another knee problem that affects young people is osteochondritis dissecans. This is a rare disorder arising in the teenage years. It is characterized by the loss of a particular segment of bone, typically of one or more femoral condyles. The cause of this disorder is unknown. The bony fragment, poorly fixed to the underlying skeleton, often becomes painful.

Cases often show up before a young person stops growing, usually by age twenty. When it affects adults, the problem can cause instability of the fragments. Bone fragments break free and lodge randomly within the knee, causing painful locking episodes. Significant portions of the adjoining surface may be lost eventually, resulting in arthritis.

Little league games, sports, and other routine play can generate bruises and fractures around the knee.

Communicating with Kids

Lastly, kids will be kids, and their knees have more contact with the ground than most adults. Ask any mom about the grass stains on the knees of their kids' pants, or how many pairs of pants get thrown out because of holes in the knees.

Here we come to the parental factor. Many parents may want their children to be active, sometimes participating in more than one sport a season. Sometimes the kids won't oblige. Vague complaints of knee pain exempt them from competition, which can be worrisome to parents and coaches. The message is not always clear. As parents and doctors, we must learn to listen to kids closely. Is the child signaling a physical ailment, or simply a disinterest in sports? Sometimes we search for a physical cause when none exists. In the final analysis, remember that children rarely suffer from missing a given sports season. Be sure to investigate, but have an open mind about the analysis.

Because kids may differ in how they communicate about pain, those with pain in the knee area—especially after a fall or traumatic event, like being hit by a baseball—should be seen by a physician.

Pre-Patellar Bursitis

Pre-patellar bursitis involves the bursae sacs on the front of the kneecap. Bursae are fluid-filled sacs that are found throughout the body in areas where the skin must glide over bones. They help to minimize friction. One of the jobs of bursae in the knee is to enable the kneecap to move about freely underneath the skin. When pressure is placed on the knee from either a direct blow or from kneeling repetitively, problems can arise.

For example, this problem in the past was also called "housemaid's knees," because often those women who scrubbed floors on hands and knees suffered from this knee problem. Similarly, brick masons, carpet layers, and electricians are also afflicted. At times the condition occurs when the bursal sac becomes infected, often for reasons which are not readily apparent. Regardless of the cause of inflammation, pain and swelling can be present in front of the kneecap.

A rubbery, bulging mass in front of the kneecap that may feel sore and tender, can develop. Except in the case of infection, treatment consists of relieving pressure. Kneeling is avoided or only performed with knee pads. The good news: only in persistent cases is surgery necessary.

Plica Syndrome

Plica are normal folds of the joint capsule within the knee. However, with activities such as running and cycling, which require repetitive bending of the knee, they may chafe so extensively against the femur that soreness results. The medial plica, which is relatively large, is the one most likely to be troublesome. When this plica is irritated, there can be kneecap pain without associated swelling.

Typically the pain is tied to activity and how aggressively it is performed. In some cases, it can vanish with periods of rest. One of the problems with diagnosing this problem is that plicae cannot be seen on X-ray, and therefore the syndrome is often difficult to substantiate. And, because symptoms associated with plica syndrome are similar to other knee problems, it can be easily misdiagnosed. Treatment consists of rest or the use of anti-inflammatory medicine.

Coming Up Next

This list of knee problems is by no means exhaustive. The complexity of the knee can lead to numerous problems, with many conditions occurring in tandem.

By now, you've probably noticed that knee problems share many of the same symptoms. Our goal in the following chapters is to clear up as much confusion as possible, and help you to get the proper treatment for whatever is ailing your knee. If it turns out to be something requiring a doctor's help, we've got tips on finding the best doctor for your individual needs.

In the next chapter you will learn how to diagnose what may have gone wrong with your knee. If you can't figure it out on your own, you will at least have a good understanding of the diagnostic tests and exam that will be done in the doctor's office.

Amazingly, many times doctor visits can be confusing and intimidating. You may be poked, prodded, and at the end of it all, the doctor may use complicated terms that mean nothing to you.

All too often, a patient can leave the exam room and be asked, "Well, what did the doctor say was wrong with your knee?" The patient may display a blank look and respond with "I'm not sure." Be sure you know exactly what the doctor thinks is wrong with your knee, whether it is a bone problem, ligament problem, tendon problem, meniscus problem, or cartilage problem.

As you read through this chapter, use the blank question and answer pages at the end of this book to jot down specific questions for your doctor during your visit. We've included a few basic ones to get you started. During your visit, bring this book so the doctor can use the medical illustrations to circle or draw arrows to specific knee components. Dog ear the pages that relate to your problem. Remember, you are paying for the doctor's time. Make the best use of it.

Chapter 4

Diagnosing Knee Pain:
What Do Various Symptoms Mean?

When does knee pain spell trouble? Are clicks, catches, grinding, and pops signs of disaster? And when do you need a doctor? When can you manage with a "wait and see" approach?

Americans are a self-reliant people. Just look at the success of Home Depot. There is a certain gratification in learning how to do something yourself. When it comes to knee pain, many people self-diagnose, and then self-treat, often with incomplete or incorrect information.

Which Symptoms Are Significant?

Does your knee crack and click as your leg goes through a range of movements? If so, you may be worried that it is broken. Sound alone is a bad indicator of trouble. Provided there is no accompanying swelling or pain, clicking sounds are typically harmless.

Pain can also be misleading. Sometimes a knee with a serious problem has little or no associated pain, while a relatively healthy knee may display troubling signals following something as routine as a change in weather.

Serious Knee Symptoms

Generally speaking, the *intensity of pain* and *how rapidly it comes on*, are good indicators of the severity of a knee problem, and the need to seek care. Extreme knee pain after falling down, or hearing a pop from your knee area, could mean a fracture or torn anterior cruciate ligament. We will deal with the most serious symptoms and situations first.

Fractures

Fractures are the most typical injury to require a trip to the emergency room. Whether the result of sports or a vehicular accident, these typically require immediate care. A fracture may extend horizontally across the bone or spiral down its length. At times the bone breaks into many parts; these are labeled comminuted fractures.

Often the fracture fragments remain in normal alignment with each other. These are called non-displaced fractures, meaning that the bone is broken but remains in its proper position. On the other hand, there are displaced fractures in which the bony fragments have broken apart and fall out of alignment, often distorting the shape of the leg.

These fractures have to be "reduced" and often are immobilized with a cast. At times, because of the number of fracture fragments or tenuousness of the reduction, fractures require surgery. The orthopedic surgeon makes an incision, takes hold of the bony fragments and manipulates them back into position, typically securing them with a rod or plate and screws.

Finally there are "open" fractures. Not only is the bone fractured, but the overlying skin is cut. This opening in the skin lets in dirt and bacteria. Without prompt treatment, infection may occur.

The two most disastrous types of fractures are spiral fractures, where extreme rotational twisting has created a break line that goes up and around the bone like a spiral staircase, and comminuted fractures. Comminuted fractures are the worst possible kind of fracture. They often happen when the knee is slammed into a dashboard in a car accident, causing the bone to shatter into many pieces. In some cases, the leg might be saved in complex surgery where a metal rod called an intramedullary nail is used to reconstruct the leg and retain its same length.

For simple fractures, the doctor may perform "closed reduction," in which the bone is manipulated back into proper placement without an incision through the skin, and then a cast or brace is used to immobilize the leg while it heals. For nondisplaced fractures, no reduction may be needed before the leg is immobilized.

Complex fractures may require "open reduction," in which an orthopedic surgeon makes an incision in the leg, and during surgery manually repositions the bones into proper position so they can heal correctly.

Ligament Tears

Sensing or actually hearing a loud pop after coming down from a rebound on the basketball court or pivoting on the soccer field often indicates a torn anterior cruciate ligament.

Similarly, a blow to the outside of the knee can tear the medial collateral ligament. A direct blow to the flexed knee which often occurs in a vehicular accident can rupture a posterior cruciate ligament.

Ligament tears cause immediate pain coupled with a sensation of instability, which typically causes an individual to fall to the ground and remain there for several minutes. On arising and attempting to walk, individuals note a "wobbly" sense from within the knee and often require assistance reaching the sidelines. Swelling occurs promptly. Whether or not they are inclined to go to the emergency room immediately, those afflicted will soon end up in the doctor's office.

Tendon Problems

Most tendon problems have recurring symptoms. Patella tendinitis is typically associated with chronic pain, which surfaces during activity and resolves with rest. Soreness is noted directly at the lower end of the kneecap or at the point where the patellar tendon connects to the shin. Patellar tendinitis is painful, but typically not debilitating. For example, a six-time Grand Slam tennis player, Stefan Edberg, suffered patellar tendinitis over much of his career.

The situation is different with patellar or quadriceps tendon rupture. Typically, this occurs with a severe injury such as a sudden fall on the flexed knee. The individual experiences extreme pain and cannot actively straighten the knee. Swelling occurs promptly. Tenderness and often a visible gap at the site of the rupture is noted.

In rarer cases, the patellar tendon can tear after a particularly nasty fall or abrupt lateral movement. If this is the case, the person will be completely unable to straighten the leg, because the patellar tendon acts as the main rubber band that goes from the front of the shin to the kneecap and then to the femur so the leg can straighten. When that rubber band breaks, there is no way to straighten the leg. Like a torn quadriceps tendon, the only way back is through surgery to reconnect the tendon to its anchor point or stitch it together.

Meniscal Damage

Imagine that you have a four-wheel-drive Jeep. As it bounces down a rocky road, shock absorbers are busy minimizing the impact of the wheels on the chassis. Similarly, the knee's internal shock absorbers, the lateral and medial menisci pads, absorb much of the abuse from our weight slamming down upon our knee joints. Now, consider how hard the Jeep's shock absorbers need to work when the Jeep is hauling excess weight. It's no different with our bodies. The heavier we are, the greater the impact on those meniscus pads. Age also has its effect. By the fifth decade of our lives, one in four persons suffer a meniscal tear.

An abrupt twist of the femur on the tibia can tear a meniscus. Medial are more common than lateral meniscal tears. Pain occurs over the meniscus at the joint line. Swelling occurs with activity, and a recurrent painful sensation of catching or locking is common. If you tear a meniscus, you will notice a gradual onset of pain and swelling that worsens with activity, especially running.

Joint Problems

While the meniscus pads act as shock absorbers underneath the femur bone, the bottom of the femur bone and the top of the tibia (shin bone), as well as the inside of the kneecap have a polished surface that acts like a chrome finish on a trailer hitch. This articular cartilage enables the knee joint mechanism to glide easily. When this chrome finish is damaged, usually over time, the joint doesn't glide as easily as it should, and that's when a host of joint problems can appear.

If you want to see how articular cartilage works, next time you are getting a chicken ready to throw on the barbecue, pull apart the drumstick from the thigh bone and note the smooth surface end of the drumstick. Compare that to the dull finish of the rest of the bone. The top of your tibia, the bottom of your femur and the inside part of your kneecap have the same white, shiny, smooth surface.

Now take a knife and scrape away part of the cartilage. You will feel roughness. Consider how this roughness would impact the other moving pieces within the joint. Sometimes that roughness can come on with arthritis, a disease which reduces the smoothness of those surfaces. In a sense, arthritis is like rust. It causes added friction and eventual wear and tear on all the moving parts.

How a Doctor Diagnoses Knee Problems

A knee doctor can determine the cause of your knee problem and how to best treat it through several procedures.

The doctor visit is composed of two separate parts: questioning of the patient to develop a "patient history," and then a hands-on exam where the doctor manipulates the knee in various and precise ways to determine what the source of the problem may be.

1. The medical history

The medical history may include your family as well as your personal story. The reason a doctor asks questions about your siblings or parents is to determine whether inherited conditions, such as arthritis, exist within the family. If so, you may be prone to the same problem.

You will be asked questions about how and when you first noticed pain in your knee. This part of the exam may seem tedious, but your answers are crucial. For example, if you reveal that your knee pain occurred precisely when you came down from a rebound and you heard a loud pop . . . the doctor will have a high degree of confidence that you probably tore your anterior cruciate ligament.

On the other hand, if you explain that your knee pain gradually worsened over several years, the doctor may be led to a much different diagnosis, possibly arthritis.

The doctor may also ask if you are taking any medications or pills which might create problems. For example, steroid use can create problems with the micro circulation of the knee joint. So can the excessive use of alcohol.

Be sure to tell your doctor if you have suffered from fever or if you've noticed aches and pains in other parts of your body. For example: Is your other knee sore as well? Lyme disease, which is transmitted by a deer tick, can cause such generalized joint soreness. So can rheumatoid arthritis, or even strep throat, or the flu.

2. The hands-on knee exam

While a person can simulate or imitate the motions in the knee exam pictured in the following pages, we don't encourage you to perform it on yourself. Each maneuver that the knee specialist performs reveals something *only* to the doctor who has done thousands of such exams.

In addition, some of these maneuvers can be painful. The best reason for demonstrating them is to give insight into which tests a doctor may perform, and why he or she is twisting your leg.

3. X-rays

Decades ago, X-rays were all an orthopedic surgeon had to peer into the knee. Even today they are a crucial part of a work-up, as they can reveal fractures and a narrowing of the joint space,

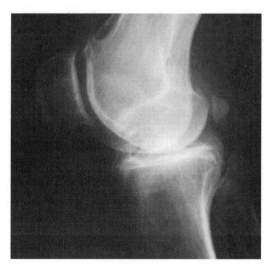

which indicates arthritis. With that said, there are some stress fractures that are so small they will not show up on X-rays. If the doctor suspects a stress fracture, he or she may order an MRI, which is a more precise diagnostic test.

On the X-ray below, for example, compare the healthy left knee and the damaged right knee. As you can see, the right knee has a smaller space between the top of the tibia (shin bone) and the bottom of the femur (thigh bone). This narrowing indicates that the shock-absorbing cartilage has worn away, leaving bone on bone contact, an advanced stage of arthritis.

X-rays are extremely limited in that they only show the bones clearly. Soft tissues like muscles, tendons, ligaments, or meniscus are very poorly seen.

4. MRI and CT Scans

Unlike X-rays that only show bones clearly, magnetic resonance imaging (MRI) scans reveal the soft tissues, such as

X-ray of an abnormal knee joint (patient's right leg)

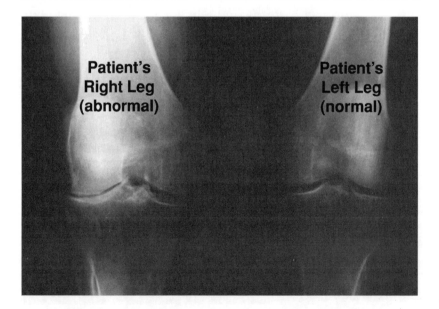

Patient's
Right Leg
(abnormal)

Patient's
Left Leg
(normal)

the meniscus and tendons. They go beyond the X-ray in what they demonstrate but, because of cost, are used sparingly.

Unlike X-rays, MRI uses the power of magnetic fields to draw images of the internal structures of the body. MRI is a relatively safe test, and in fact, safer than most tests which use radiation. However, a person undergoing an MRI must remain very still for an extended period while the computer is creating the image.

Those undergoing full body MRIs may find it uncomfortable if they have confinement anxiety because it is like laying in a very narrow tunnel. Leg and arm scans do not present this problem. For greater comfort, most knee centers will have an open MRI which is less confining and specifically designed for studies of the arm or leg, instead of the entire body.

MRI of the knee joint, side view

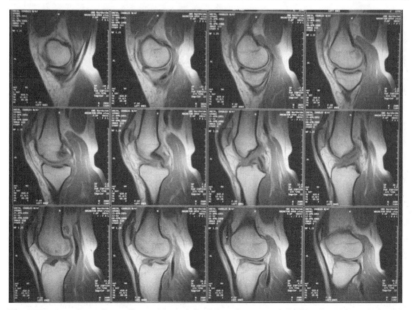

The MRI scan above shows the position of the femur, kneecap, and tibia. Several scans in this series reveal the meniscus pads. By viewing them, the doctor can examine these shock-absorbing menisci pads to see if they are torn.

5. Diagnostic treatments

In a sense, "diagnostic treatments" may sound like contradictory terms. But there are certain "treatments" that a doctor may try. If they succeed, they may confirm a doctor's suspicions about the cause of your pain. This can include use of oral medications to reduce inflammation, draining fluid, or injections into the knee joint.

MRI scan, axial view of the knee

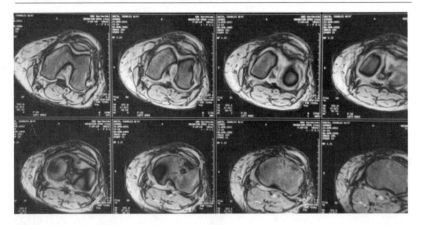

In the past, physicians would have to do surgery to see the soft tissues inside the knee. Now a painless MRI scan can take a picture of the inside of the knee. Each MRI diagnostic test will provide the doctor with a dozen or more freeze-frame images of the knee from various sidecut views, as if a saw sliced through the knee. Each frame represents a different position, as if the slice were a couple millimeters higher than the previous scan. The MRI scan above show sidecut views of the interior knee space, as if you were looking directly down on the top of the tibia.

Peering inside the knee and repairing the knee

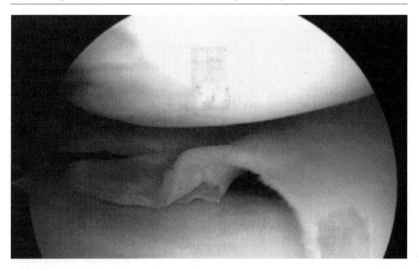

Above left is a torn meniscus, with the tear visible at the far left of the image. Below, the surgeon has removed the torn part of the meniscus leaving as much healthy meniscus as possible.

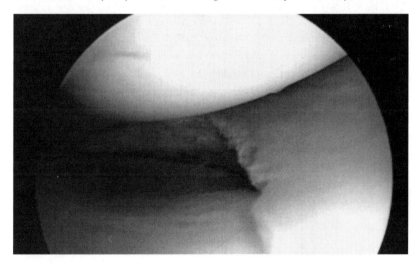

Peering inside the knee and repairing the knee

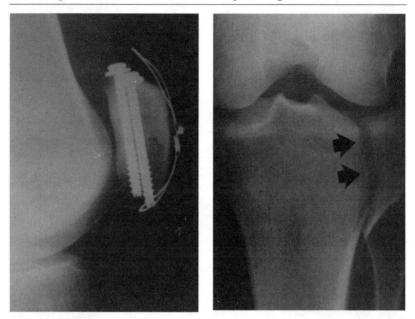

Above left is an X-ray after surgery of a fracture of the patella (kneecap) that is held together with screws and a wire. Above right shows a fractured tibial plateau suffered from a skiing accident. Below right shows a healthy ACL under arthroscopy.

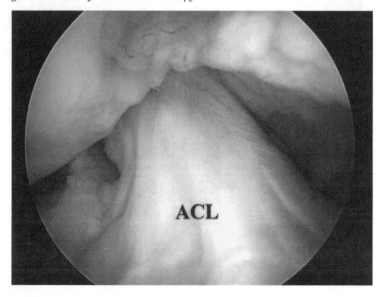

6. Arthroscopy

One tool, both diagnostic and surgical, which has dramatically improved knee care is the arthroscope. Years ago, if a surgeon needed to inspect the knee he or she would have to make a long incision to enter and visually explore the site. Unfortunately, this incision damaged soft tissues and slowed rehabilitation. The arthroscope changed that. Instead of a three-inch inci-

Arthroscopy of the knee to repair torn meniscus

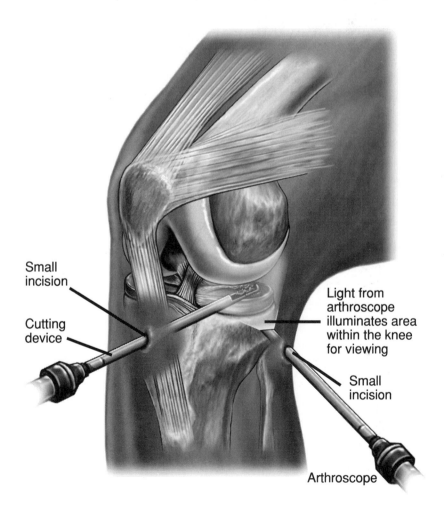

Small incision

Cutting device

Light from arthroscope illuminates area within the knee for viewing

Small incision

Arthroscope

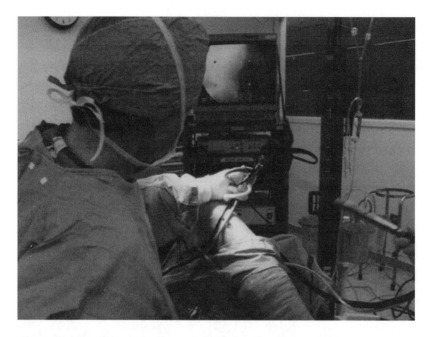

Shown above, the arthroscope involves several tools including an external TV screen and a long, hollow tube with an attached camera, which transmits a picture to the TV screen. Inside the knee joint, the surgeon maneuvers the camera tool to reveal the entire knee. A probe is introduced through a second hole to allow structures to be touched and manipulated.

sion, knee surgery is now done through small puncture incisions about one to two mm in length. Rehabilitation is rapid, and patients return to activity faster. Currently, more than 90 percent of routine knee surgery is done with an arthroscope.

Previously, when MRI was not available, it was common for surgeons to perform exploratory surgery, to locate the cause of the problem. Nowadays, with MRI, the doctor typically has a good idea of what is wrong before proceeding with arthroscopy.

Time for a Visit to the Knee Doctor

Okay, let's head for the doctor's office to see how a knee exam is performed. On the following pages you will learn the motions that will be used to evaluate your knee.

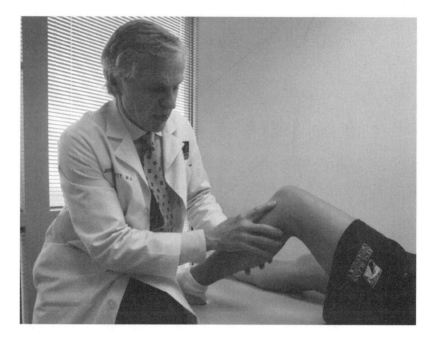

1 *Okay, where does it hurt?*

Where EXACTLY does it hurt? Your knee doctor will need to know. As shown in the pictures above and below, the doctor may press, poke, and prod various areas around the knee. Your grimace or yelp is key to determining the correct diagnosis. In the picture above, pressing on the lateral collateral ligament may reveal pain. If so, it may imply a torn lateral collateral ligament. On the right, pressure around the kneecap area can reveal if the patellar tendon is particularly sensitive. Patellar tendinitis is typically just a problem of overuse.

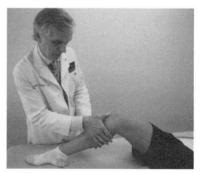

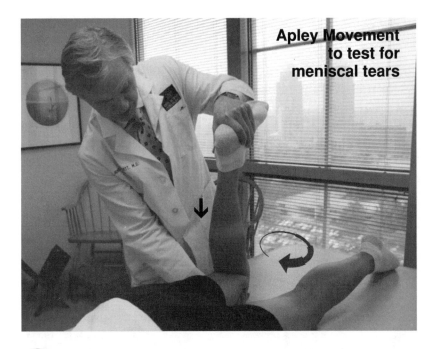

Apley Movement to test for meniscal tears

2 *Tests that reveal if the shock-absorbing meniscus is torn*

There are also specific motions that can help the knee specialist determine if a meniscus is damaged.

If you imagine your femur resting on two circular-shaped shock-absorbing donuts that sit atop your tibia, twisting of the tibia can cause a grinding sensation, which may imply that the meniscus is damaged. Pain on rotation, for instance, can imply a meniscal tear of either the lateral (outer) meniscus or medial (inner) meniscus.

Using the Apley Test, shown above, the doctor holds the leg and applies pressure on the foot which transfers pressure on the knee joint, and then twists to test for joint play.

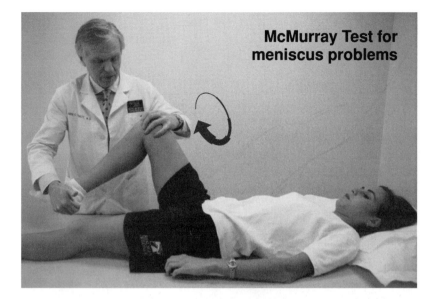

**McMurray Test for
meniscus problems**

The McMurray Test, shown above, has the patient lying on her back while the knee specialist bends the knee, past ninety degrees. While straightening the leg, the knee specialist twists the knee, feeling along the joint line for pops, clicks, or grinding. In a sense, it's much like a carpenter testing a door hinge by closing and opening it to listen for squeaks.

Since a healthy knee can also sometimes make suspicious noises, it's important to rely on a knee specialist to interpret such noises. The sounds and sensations related to the knee are only informative to the knee specialist who can interpret these sensations in the context of thousands of other knee exams already performed over years of professional practice.

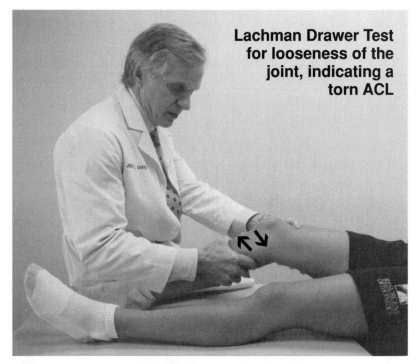

**Lachman Drawer Test
for looseness of the
joint, indicating a
torn ACL**

 Tests that reveal which ligament may be injured

The knee doctor can determine which ligament may be damaged through several movements which will reveal excessive movement. The Lachman Test is one of several movements that enables the knee doctor to check for a torn ACL.

When you consider the specific roles of the various ligaments, you can begin to understand the rationale for the various maneuvers. The medial collateral ligament limits how much the leg can bend outward. On the other hand, the lateral collateral ligament controls and limits how much the leg can bend inward.

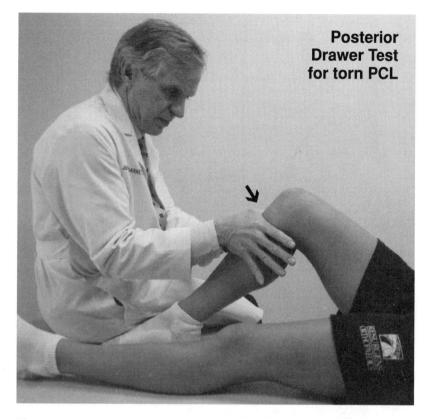

Posterior Drawer Test for torn PCL

The Posterior Drawer Test enables the knee specialist to check for looseness in the joint. In the Posterior Drawer Test, the doctor pushes the leg downward like closing a drawer. A knee with a torn PCL may move up to one-half inch. Overall, the damaged joint may appear dramatically looser than the other, healthy knee.

Tests that reveal if the ACL is torn

Shown below are the Pivot Shift Test and the Anterior Drawer Test. The doctor grabs the lower leg, braces the knee, and tries to raise the shin bone upward to see if the ACL rubber band is excessively loose.

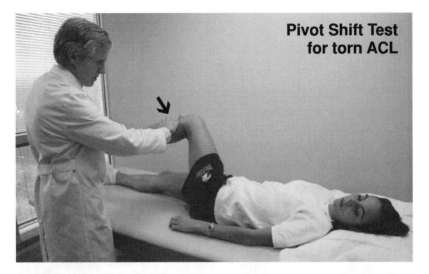

Pivot Shift Test for torn ACL

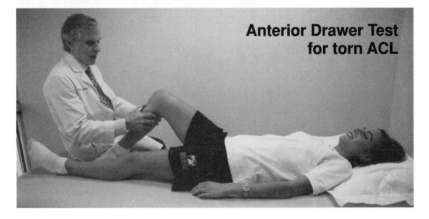

Anterior Drawer Test for torn ACL

Symptom Flow Charts for Self-Diagnosis

The following pages show several flow charts which can help check specific symptoms against possible diagnoses. The first chart relates to knee problems which begin abruptly, often after an accident. The second chart covers knee problems which develop over days, weeks, or months.

Later in this chapter, you will find a summary that outlines the most common symptoms and their causes, treatments, and recovery time. This will help gauge expectations about the time required for rehabilitation.

ACUTE KNEE PAIN: Flow Chart for Self-Diagnosis

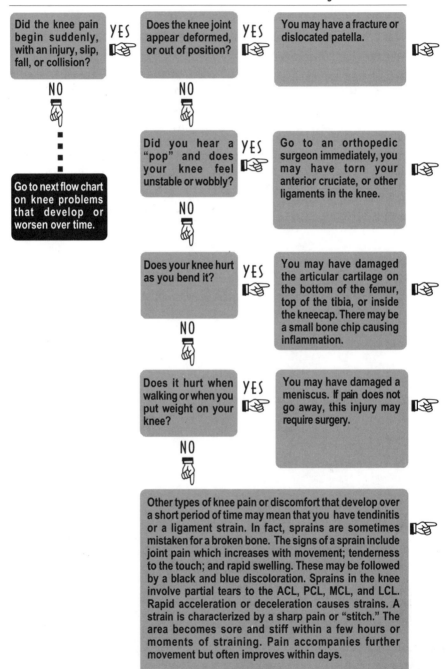

Did the knee pain begin suddenly, with an injury, slip, fall, or collision? **YES** ☞

NO ☟

Go to next flow chart on knee problems that develop or worsen over time.

Does the knee joint appear deformed, or out of position? **YES** ☞

NO ☟

You may have a fracture or dislocated patella. ☞

Did you hear a "pop" and does your knee feel unstable or wobbly? **YES** ☞

NO ☟

Go to an orthopedic surgeon immediately, you may have torn your anterior cruciate, or other ligaments in the knee. ☞

Does your knee hurt as you bend it? **YES** ☞

NO ☟

You may have damaged the articular cartilage on the bottom of the femur, top of the tibia, or inside the kneecap. There may be a small bone chip causing inflammation. ☞

Does it hurt when walking or when you put weight on your knee? **YES** ☞

NO ☟

You may have damaged a meniscus. If pain does not go away, this injury may require surgery. ☞

Other types of knee pain or discomfort that develop over a short period of time may mean that you have tendinitis or a ligament strain. In fact, sprains are sometimes mistaken for a broken bone. The signs of a sprain include joint pain which increases with movement; tenderness to the touch; and rapid swelling. These may be followed by a black and blue discoloration. Sprains in the knee involve partial tears to the ACL, PCL, MCL, and LCL. Rapid acceleration or deceleration causes strains. A strain is characterized by a sharp pain or "stitch." The area becomes sore and stiff within a few hours or moments of straining. Pain accompanies further movement but often improves within days. ☞

... & Self-Help/First-Aid Flow Chart

STOP 👉 Stop what you are doing immediately and go to a hospital emergency room or an orthopedic surgeon specializing in knee problems.

🚑 If possible, splint the leg to limit the movement of the knee until you reach the doctor. Do not put any weight on the knee. Use a wheelchair, a cane, or crutch to prevent putting any weight on the leg, which might cause further damage to the joint.

STOP 👉 Stop what you are doing. Continuing activity despite the feeling that the knee is unstable can cause additional damage to other ligaments, meniscus, and cartilage. Try ice on the knee to control swelling. Take anti-inflammatories like Advil or Nuprin until your doctor's appointment. About a third of ligament tears get better with exercises, a third may need a brace, and a third may need surgery. (See ACL repair.)

STOP 👉 Try anti-inflammatories, as directed on the bottle, for two days to reduce the chronic inflammation.

Restrict activity which causes pain. Call a specialist for a more in-depth diagnosis and treatment.

STOP 👉 Try anti-inflammatories, as directed on the bottle, for two days to reduce the chronic inflammation.

Call a knee specialist. A serious meniscus tear can require surgery.

STOP

Use R•I•C•E
for sore knees

R: Rest
I: Ice
C: Compression
E: Elevation

👉 Try anti-inflammatories to reduce the chronic inflammation. Also, use ice to reduce swelling.

The good news is that many knee injuries are simply strains from overuse. The three knee tendons at risk for pain are the patellar tendon, the quadriceps tendon, and the popliteus. Dancers, cyclists, and runners frequently experience bouts of tendinitis, when heavy usage stretches out their tendons. This can include patellar tendinitis or patellofemeral pain syndrone. Neither requires surgery. When you return to activity, keep in mind that in sports like tennis, strains are often caused by poor footwork. Consider a tennis lesson with a pro who can improve your preparation and anticipation so there is less need for lunging and uncoordinated stops and starts.

CHRONIC KNEE PAIN: Flow Chart for Self-Diagnosis

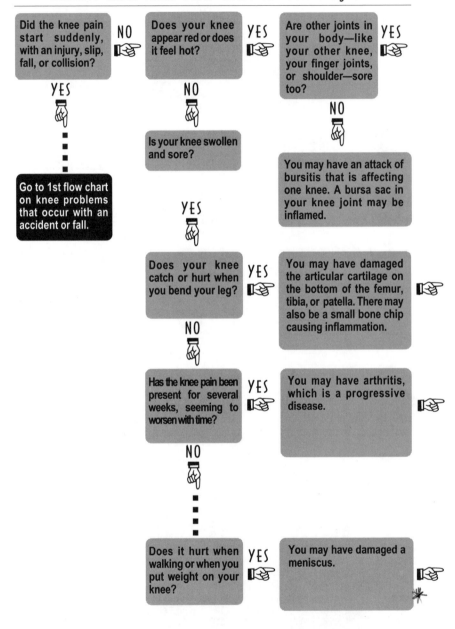

Did the knee pain start suddenly, with an injury, slip, fall, or collision?

NO 👉

YES 👇

Go to 1st flow chart on knee problems that occur with an accident or fall.

Does your knee appear red or does it feel hot?

YES 👉

NO 👇

Is your knee swollen and sore?

YES 👇

Does your knee catch or hurt when you bend your leg?

YES 👉

NO 👇

Has the knee pain been present for several weeks, seeming to worsen with time?

YES 👉

NO 👇

Does it hurt when walking or when you put weight on your knee?

YES 👉

Are other joints in your body—like your other knee, your finger joints, or shoulder—sore too?

YES 👉

NO 👇

You may have an attack of bursitis that is affecting one knee. A bursa sac in your knee joint may be inflamed.

You may have damaged the articular cartilage on the bottom of the femur, tibia, or patella. There may also be a small bone chip causing inflammation. 👉

You may have arthritis, which is a progressive disease. 👉

You may have damaged a meniscus. 👉

... & Self Help/First-Aid

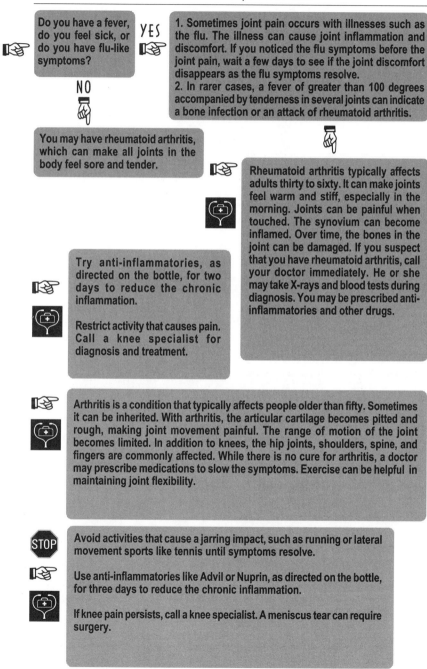

Do you have a fever, do you feel sick, or do you have flu-like symptoms?

YES

1. Sometimes joint pain occurs with illnesses such as the flu. The illness can cause joint inflammation and discomfort. If you noticed the flu symptoms before the joint pain, wait a few days to see if the joint discomfort disappears as the flu symptoms resolve.

2. In rarer cases, a fever of greater than 100 degrees accompanied by tenderness in several joints can indicate a bone infection or an attack of rheumatoid arthritis.

NO

You may have rheumatoid arthritis, which can make all joints in the body feel sore and tender.

Rheumatoid arthritis typically affects adults thirty to sixty. It can make joints feel warm and stiff, especially in the morning. Joints can be painful when touched. The synovium can become inflamed. Over time, the bones in the joint can be damaged. If you suspect that you have rheumatoid arthritis, call your doctor immediately. He or she may take X-rays and blood tests during diagnosis. You may be prescribed anti-inflammatories and other drugs.

Try anti-inflammatories, as directed on the bottle, for two days to reduce the chronic inflammation.

Restrict activity that causes pain. Call a knee specialist for diagnosis and treatment.

Arthritis is a condition that typically affects people older than fifty. Sometimes it can be inherited. With arthritis, the articular cartilage becomes pitted and rough, making joint movement painful. The range of motion of the joint becomes limited. In addition to knees, the hip joints, shoulders, spine, and fingers are commonly affected. While there is no cure for arthritis, a doctor may prescribe medications to slow the symptoms. Exercise can be helpful in maintaining joint flexibility.

STOP

Avoid activities that cause a jarring impact, such as running or lateral movement sports like tennis until symptoms resolve.

Use anti-inflammatories like Advil or Nuprin, as directed on the bottle, for three days to reduce the chronic inflammation.

If knee pain persists, call a knee specialist. A meniscus tear can require surgery.

SYMPTOM / CAUSE

Symptom	Probable cause
Pain, accompanied by a loud pop from the knee area, followed by a feeling of instability in the knee. Symptoms that result from a twisting injury.	Torn anterior cruciate ligament.
Inability to straighten the leg from a fall onto the knee or a direct blow to the kneecap.	Fracture around the kneecap area.
Abrupt pain at the inner or outer part of the knee accompanied by a feeling of instability in the knee. This is caused by a blow to the outer part of the knee, possibly from football, basketball, soccer, or other contact sport.	A blow to the inner side of the knee may have torn the lateral collateral ligament. A blow to the outer side of the knee may have torn the medial collateral ligament.
Fall on a flexed knee. Unable to extend the leg.	Torn quadriceps or patellar tendon.

TREATMENT / RECOVERY TIME NEEDED

Treatment	Recovery time needed
A fully torn ACL requires surgery to return stability to the knee joint. Partially torn ACLs might heal with time and special exercises to some extent without surgery.	ACL surgery requires six weeks to return to moderate activities. Return to sports requiring cutting maneuvers takes five to six months.
If there is a fracture, surgery may be required.	Fractures can require three to six months for recovery.
An isolated tear of the MCL or LCL does not require surgery.	Recovery from a torn MCL or LCL takes one to two months. Afterward, the knee joint can be almost as strong as before the injury.
Tears of the quadriceps or patellar tendon require surgery.	Recovery takes six to twelve months.

Some Common Questions

1. If the problem is related to overuse, (i.e., tendinitis or a stress fracture) must I stop exercising?

Most individuals who train to the point of overtaxing their limbs, typically are doing so for a reason. Emotionally, athletes may be strongly bound to their goals and training programs. However, common sense dictates that to cure an overuse problem there has to be, if not cessation of activity, at least a lessening of its intensity.

For a distance runner this means reducing the number of miles run, or cross training with cycling or swimming. Don't be surprised if you find yourself obsessed with your goals and training habits. You may be far too rigid in your approach to fitness. Except for Olympians, most individuals can give up one training session for a race, however special it may seem at the time. Use common sense.

2. If I am overweight and my knees are becoming arthritic, must I lose weight or may I simply exercise and use anti-inflammatory medication?

Maintenance of reasonable body weight by balancing proper diet and exercise can be difficult. Many Americans weigh far too much, much to their detriment.

The situation is often aggravated by external pressures. For instance, stress from extended hours at work often leads to a poor diet. Similarly, depression can lead to overeating. However, to keep your knees from wearing out prematurely, losing those extra pounds is important.

3. The doctor tells me that I have a torn cartilage. Is it imperative that I undergo surgery?

Unless you have a "locked knee," the need for arthroscopic surgery to resect a torn piece of cartilage is a matter of relative necessity. Rarely is it an emergency.

The question you must *ask the doctor* is how significant is the tear. The question you must *ask yourself* is how much does it hurt or interfere with activity.

If a tear is small, or if you suffer little or no pain, the decision to operate can be postponed. As weeks or months progress, you can judge the need for the operation for yourself. However, if a tear is large and you are swollen or suffer recurrent bouts of locking, then the answer is obvious. You have a mechanical problem which needs mechanical, i.e., surgical solution.

4. *I have recently injured my knee. An MRI scan revealed a complete tear of the anterior cruciate ligament. Do I need surgery?*

Given a tear of the anterior cruciate ligament, the need for surgery is generally based on a patient's athletic profile irrespective of age or gender. For instance, an eighteen-year-old high school soccer player will probably need anterior cruciate ligament reconstruction. So will a thirty-five-year-old housewife who plays A level tennis. Neither age or gender has any bearing. If active, even a sixty-year-old may require surgery. However, if an individual's athletic spectrum encompasses more than jogging, cycling, or swimming, that is, if they do not participate in jumping or cutting activities, cruciate ligament reconstruction is probably unnecessary.

5. *I am an active athlete and understand that I require anterior cruciate ligament reconstruction. One doctor has recommended reconstruction with a portion of patellar tendon graft, the second recommended a hamstring graft. Which should I choose?*

The first decision with anterior cruciate ligament injury is whether you need surgery. The second is which graft would be appropriate.

Luckily in this day and age, it is difficult to demonstrate differences between patellar tendon and hamstring graft. In most instances, both will yield strong graft material for a successful reconstruction. However, some doctors only perform one type of reconstruction.

There is indeed a bias toward utilizing the patellar tendon reconstruction for the larger individual with a more strenuous athletic activity, i.e., the professional football player or college basketball player. However, a hamstring reconstruction is less painful and associated with a more rapid rehabilitation. Also, it is typically more acceptable to the middle-aged athlete seeking to minimize discomfort and lost work time.

6. *I am a sixty-year-old. My knees are swollen and hurt every day. Do I need total knee replacement?*

The decision as to whether to proceed with total knee replacement depends upon a variety of factors. The first question to ask is to what extent does pain impede your lifestyle. Does it influence your ability to work, maintain a household, or enjoy yourself?

If the symptoms are annoying but tolerable, then the answer is clear—irrespective of what X-rays show—you don't need knee replacements yet.

The second question which you must ask yourself is whether you have exhausted all self-help measures. For example, ask yourself the following questions and answer honestly:

1. Have you reduced body weight?
2. Are you exercising to keep your legs strong?
3. Have you used anti-inflammatory medication to reduce pain?
4. In moments of crisis have you tried a shot of cortisone?
5. Can or are you willing to make some modification in your lifestyle?

If these factors have not been considered as yet, then you probably have some work to do before asking a surgeon to replace your knee.

Part 3

Treatment

Chapter 5

How You Can Treat Some Knee Problems without Surgery

Our objective in this chapter is to help you recover without surgery. Remember: Of all injured knees, typically 80 percent will not need surgery. That's promising news.

With that said, if you heard a loud pop when your anterior cruciate ligament snapped last week while playing basketball, or if you have a fracture as a result of a car accident, it's likely that the strategies in this chapter will not be of much value to you. Anytime there is a *severe* structural break, tear, or deterioration, you may need the help of a surgeon to repair the damage.

In your battle back to activity, keep in mind that perserverance and overall fitness will be key allies. It can be tough to do knee exercises and stay fit when you have sore knees. Once your doctor has confirmed that exercises will not further damage your knees, and that specialized exercises are the best prescription for you, do whatever you can to latch onto positive roles models to keep you focused on successful rehabilitation.

Also keep in mind that your objective may not be to get back to such a high level of fitness. Unlike Steffi Graf, who put in an incredible effort to come back after two years worth of knee pain to win the French Open in 1999, you are not trying to get your knees to carry you to a Grand Slam tennis final in Paris.

If you have knee pain or a serious knee problem, adjust your expectations so you can focus on how far you are getting instead of how far you still need to go. Set realistic and practical goals.

In the chapter that features ACL repair, Kevin's goal was to first get back to playing and enjoying golf. Next, he hopes to work back up to tennis, which is far more demanding on his knees. By adjusting to an easier activity level, Kevin gives his knees a chance to gain strength from all the walking associated with golf and the lessened rotational stress of the golf swing. Another issue to consider during your knee rehabilitation is to change your focus from pain to activity. If you continually focus on the soreness in your knees, it will be difficult to stay with your exercises and your activities.

For example, Stefan Edberg—winner of six Grand Slam singles titles—was regarded as one of the best ever at serve and volley tennis, something that requires tremendous knee bending and fast lateral movement. It is a little known fact that Edberg suffered from patellar tendinitis for most of his career. He never complained of it. And even as his career trailed off in his late twenties, he never used knee pain as a reason for his retirement. Years later, after his retirement from competitive tennis, Edberg stayed active by playing tennis with Tim Henman, a top ten serve and volleyer who was trying to emulate Edberg's aggressive net play. Find your role model and source of encouragement. Then remember, your objective is probably not to get back to championship level activity, just a level that keeps you active and having fun.

About Severity of Tears, and the Ability of Certain Ligaments to Heal on Their Own

Your knee physician may categorize your ligament tear as a grade one tear, grade two tear, or grade three tear, with grade three being the worst kind of tear. Grade one tears of a ligament can be painful, but there is no instability. Grade two tears include some instability. Grade three tears have instability of five to ten millimeters in the joint. But the ligament involved can also be key to determine if you need surgery or not.

For example, hockey player Brett Hull played through three regular periods of game six of the 1999 Stanley Cup play-offs, and then three more periods during triple overtime with a torn MCL. Finally, after nearly six periods of hockey, an exhausted Hull stick-handled the puck past the Buffalo Sabres goalie to win the Stanley Cup—all with a grade three tear of his medial collateral ligament. This is not to imply that Hull will not have his MCL repaired, as he likely will find that he cannot continue without it being repaired. It is just that he made the decision to delay that surgery until he got through the career highlight of the Stanley Cup playoffs.

In his favor is that torn MCLs can sometimes heal on their own—even grade three tears. And to some extent the same can be said for torn LCLs.

That cannot be said for a torn ACL or torn PCL, however. A completely torn ACL will not heal on its own. And a torn PCL will heal with so much scar tissue that it may ultimately require surgery to fix it correctly for the long term.

Anti-Inflammatories and Medicating Yourself

Most cases of arthritis or joint pain are treated first with some sort of over-the-counter anti-inflammatory pain relievers. NSAIDs (nonsteroidal anti-inflammatory drugs) like aspirin or Tylenol, and ibuprofen pain relievers like Nuprin, Advil, or Motrin IB are used to reduce inflammation.

While these anti-inflammatories may be valuable in providing temporary pain relief and reducing inflammation, they can be harmful if taken for extended periods of time. When taken for long periods of time, they can cause ulcers and other gastrointestinal problems. Worse, they have been proven to inhibit cartilage repair.

Remember, anti-inflammatories are a short-term solution only. Relying on them on a daily basis only masks the symptoms of pain. If you have continuing pain, you should identify what is causing the problem. Your knee specialist will be able to provide the best advice for repair or long-term management of your specific knee problem.

Also, be careful to always follow the directions on the label. Just because drugs are available over the counter without a prescription does NOT mean they can't hurt you. Long term abuse of any drug can do permanent and irreversible damage to your internal organs. Excessive use of Tylenol can cause liver damage, just as aspirin can affect the lining of the stomach.

New drugs for osteoarthritis

Even new miracle drugs can have negative side effects. For instance, there is a new class of arthritis drugs known as COX-2 inhibitors. The two most popular prescription arthritis drugs of this family are Celebrex by Searle and Vioxx by Merck. Both propose to lessen stiffness, enabling the arthritis sufferer to climb stairs and do other activities of daily living with lessened pain. After its first fourteen weeks on the market, Celebrex reportedly exceeded Viagra (a pill for impotence) as one of the hottest selling new drugs on the market.

These drugs, which are helpful for arthritis, can also inhibit the body's natural ability to heal stomach ulcers. Then again, the same drugs may have some positive properties for fighting colon cancer. Generally speaking, be careful with any drug, even those over the counter. Get the advice of a doctor before you get in the habit of living on certain over-the-counter medications. You might not want to live with the long-term effect of your self- medication.

And for women who are pregnant, ALWAYS consult a doctor before taking any medication, even over the counter medications, just to be safe for your unborn baby on board.

Enzyme Supplements

Many enzymes are responsible for inflammation, but others when taken in certain doses can actually reduce inflammation before it causes damage.

The enzymes used to treat arthritis have been found to be at least as effective as the NSAIDs like aspirin or Tylenol. Enzymes have been declared by the FDA as "GRAS" (Generally Regarded as Safe), and they come in capsules that can be taken orally.

Enzymes commonly taken for arthritis or joint pain include bromelain, papain, rutin, trypsin, and chymotrysin. These specific enzymes contain anti-inflammatory properties, and they break up antigen-antibody complexes that are involved in autoimmune reactions, which aggravate conditions like rheumatoid arthritis.

Do It Yourself Physical Therapy

Remember the RICE formula for treatment of acute knee pain from activity: Rest, Ice, Compression, Elevation.

Ice can control swelling and inflammation initially. Be careful you don't overdo the contact of ice with the skin as you don't want to cause skin damage. An ice bag in a towel place around the knee is a suitable way to apply cold to the knee. Another trick is to get some Dixie cups, fill several with water, place them into the freezer. After activity, take one of the Dixie cups out, peel back its edge, and you have a nice ice applicator for your knee.

Generally speaking, most physical therapists who specialize in knee treatment spend little time in "passive modalities" like ice, heat, electrical stimulation, or ultrasound treatments. They know that the most success is gained from getting the person moving with special exercises.

Because of the significance of this area, we've dedicated an entire chapter to exercise therapy for knee problems. But first, let's continue on with other mainstream and alternative treatments for you to consider.

Orthotics and Braces

In some cases, knee pain can be alleviated by something as simple as using a foot orthotic or knee brace. Foot orthotics are orthopedic devices like insoles or supports that are usually custom fit to control the foot and correct imbalances. An orthotic foot support can raise the arch of the foot and realign the bones of the foot to prevent excess motion when you bear weight. Foot problems can sometimes cause ankle, knee, hip, and back problems.

If you are an avid runner, and you are suffering from knee problems, you may want to explore an orthotic foot device. The device could position your foot in such a way that knee pain could be alleviated. Many times, improper foot mechanics leads to improper running or other physical motion, and this can damage the knee. If you are suffering from arthritis, or you are overweight, the foot orthotic could help by repositioning your foot and counteracting stress on your knee to allow greater comfort and mobility for greater lengths of time. Orthotics come in rigid, semi-rigid, and soft materials. The rigid materials are generally prescribed when entire control and support is needed. The semi-rigid materials offer support, but they also allow for shock absorption.

Who Should You Ask About Foot Orthotics?

Orthopedic surgeons, physiatrists (specialists in physical medicine or rehabilitation), and podiatrists all specialize in musculoskeletal problems. Podiatrists specialize in only foot problems, and some are proficient in understanding how orthotics can lessen the strain on the leg joints. Physiatrists, also called PMR doctors, have advanced training in understanding gait and the mechanics involved in walking and running. All can determine which orthotic may be best for you, and if an orthotic might help relieve your knee pain.

It is important that you do not buy orthotic foot supports and begin to wear them without a doctor's consultation. Wearing improper orthotics may do more damage to your knee if they position the foot incorrectly.

About Knee Braces and Knee Support Wraps

Knee braces can be used to help an existing knee injury, or to protect the knee from future injury. Before these devices are used, you should consult with a physician. If worn improperly, the brace could do damage, and wearing it for a long period of time would not allow the muscles around your knee to grow stronger.

A study from the Surgical Clinic of the Ullevaal Hospital at the University of Oslo in Norway found that patients in their study using a knee brace after anterior cruciate ligament (ACL) reconstruction had increased thigh atrophy after wearing the brace for three months.

Said another way, using a brace is like using a crutch. While it can help you become active after an injury, depending upon it excessively doesn't encourage the supporting muscles to strengthen. And in a sense, you become dependent upon that crutch, so when it isn't there, you can have problems.

With that said, a subliminal function of a knee brace is that it can act like a string around your finger—to remind you to be careful during activity, and not be overly aggressive with the knee joint.

You should be aware that a brace is only an additional aid to medical treatment. We recommend that you first visit with a knee specialist before going out and buying a brace to wear for your knee pain. You need the source of your knee pain, and only an orthopedic surgeon can make such a diagnosis.

In many cases, the right kind of knee brace can indeed help control knee pain and the stresses placed on the knee. A study conducted by the Cincinnati Sports Medicine and Orthopedic Center in Ohio tested patients with chronic knee pain and arthrosis using a knee brace to determine whether the brace alleviated pain and increased function. Following nine weeks of wearing the brace, only 31 percent of the patients continued to have pain, compared to the 78 percent that had pain before the brace.

The center concluded that the knee brace provides short-term pain relief and improved function. For patients who can not undergo immediate surgery, it can buy additional time. And this may be a worthwhile way to go. The human body has amazing recuperative abilities, which can even surprise doctors.

If you are professional baseball player with a limited number of productive years, you may not have the luxury of taking it slow for a couple seasons to see if your knee can recuperate and heal on its own without surgery.

That's why it's common to read in the daily newspaper about athletes who have arthroscopic surgery for knee problems. They simply can't wait, because they depend on their knees for their earning power. Now, for the rest of us who are playing tennis on the weekends for recreation, we may be better off seeing if time and Mother Nature can save us from surgery.

A knee brace may also be used after surgery to improve mobility. A study conducted at the Department of Exercise and

Sport Science at East Carolina University concluded that walking while wearing a knee brace can help the knee joint and the replaced ligament after ACL reconstruction surgery.

Wrapping your knee with an Ace bandage or other tight brace intended to hold the joint or kneecap tightly in position, can also lead to problems. If the joint is wrapped or compressed tightly, blood clots could occur because the large vein behind the joint becomes blocked. But when knees develop mechanical problems, your doctor may recommend that you use a brace to support an injured ligament, control instability, or relieve pressure on a damaged component of the knee.

How Braces Work

Braces are commonly used for sprains of the medial collateral ligament. This injury requires rest. For many individuals that means cessation of activity. For those who must play, it means protecting the injured ligament from further side-to-side stress and injury. The struts on a double upright hinge brace work well in such instances, allowing many athletes to return to sport sooner.

Bracing for an ACL injury

A torn anterior cruciate ligament is a different matter. Those who suffer partial or complete tears, but decide against surgery, must depend on a brace to protect the joint during recovery.

However, it is rotatory rather than side-to-side stability which is in question. A simple upright hinge brace is inadequate. A sports brace which resists torque is necessary. These braces are called "derotation" braces and typically are customized for a given individual.

A disagreement exists as to whether such braces should be worn in the first year after anterior cruciate ligament reconstruction when the new ligament is still remolding and gaining ultimate strength. Experts are split in their opinions. Up to forty percent no longer use a brace at all, fifty percent use it for a year, and ten percent still recommend its use for a lifetime. The best way for you to decide is to consult your surgeon.

How effective are anterior cruciate ligament braces? Are they worth their high price tag? Can they predictably prevent reinjury and be used in place of surgery? In reality, no brace is perfect. Anterior cruciate or derotational braces are no exception even when customized for given patient. Why? To steady the knee, these braces must grip the soft tissues of the leg, namely the muscles of the thigh and calf. Even with a thin leg, this grip is less than perfectly secure. Under the very best of circumstances, rotatory stress may overwhelm the ability of such braces to withstand excessive torque. In conclusion, braces are helpful, but not foolproof.

Bracing for a PCL injury

Posterior cruciate ligament injuries often do not require surgery. Unfortunately, it is difficult for a brace to compensate for this type of instability, especially if there is a question of reducing the posterior sag which develops with mild to moderate ligament damage.

Bracing for a dislocated kneecap

Instability due to patellar dislocation requires a special type of brace. Rather than limit side-to-side pressure or torque, you are trying to capture the patella and hold it still while the knee flexes and extends as well as twists. But the patella is small and difficult for a brace to grasp. However, a "Palombo" brace which acts as a buttress against dislocation is often effective in preventing recurrent dislocation, thus obviating the need for surgery.

Bracing for an arthritic knee

The arthritic knee is probably the most common reason that people use a brace. A simple neoprene sleeve will yield a sense of support, help resist swelling and, at the same time, warm an injured joint. All three effects yield a sense of comfort and well-being. Adding hinged uprights to the sides helps resist side-to-side stresses common in tennis and soccer. If arthritis is limited to one side of the knee, a brace can help to unload the affected compartment. For those with medial compartment arthritis, especially those with bowed legs, an "unloader brace" which reduces pressure on the medial compartment can be very helpful.

Dieting to Reduce Knee Pain

What does dieting have to do with sore knees? A ton–literally. Around 1990, about 25 percent of Americans were overweight. At the time that had medical researchers alarmed, and they set out to reduce that number by the millennium. Unfortunately, instead of people becoming less overweight, the percentage of overweight Americans has grown. Now, half of Americans are overweight. Worse, about one in four Americans are obese. Obese is defined as a body mass index of greater than thirty. This isn't thirty pounds, but a BMI of 30, which are two different things. For example, a person five-foot-nine would have to weigh more than 200 pounds to be obese.

The Centers for Disease Control, which tracks such statistics, warns that we as a nation are facing a real epidemic of obesity. If the trend continues, medical experts warn that nearly all Americans will be overweight within two generations.

For years, medical experts have warned that being fat shortens life span. Statistics show that someone who is forty-five pounds overweight has a 165 percent greater risk of heart attack. Excess body fat also accounts for 80 percent of type II diabetes cases. Obesity also raises the risk of gallstones and arthritis. The most gruesome statistic of all is that the nation's largest casket company notes that sales of oversized coffins are up 20 percent over the last five years.

It's easy to find yourself overweight in America. We've gotten careless about how we eat. It's estimated that Americans spend about 45 percent of their food budget on meals and snacks outside the home. Someone's benefitting from that, while our knees pay the price. Consider that there are more than 200,000 fast food restaurants in the United States, with most of them offering fatty foods. Even the vegetables we eat are re-engineered in bad ways. One-third of the vegetables eaten by kids, for example, are in the form of french fries or potato chips. Also, some

Fat Lands

Percent of population that is obese, ranked by fattest men

	Men	Women
Kuwait	32.3%	40.6%
United States	**19.5%**	**25.0%**
Germany	17.2%	19.3%
England	15.0%	16.0%
Australia	11.5%	13.2%
Mexico	11.0%	23.0%
South Africa	7.9%	44.4%
Brazil	5.9%	13.3%
Sweden	5.3%	9.1%
China	0.7%	0.7%

Source: World Health Organization report 1997.
Obesity = BMI of thirty or higher. For example, a person five-foot-nine
would have to weigh more than 200 pounds to be obese.

common snacks that don't seem fattening can sneak up on us. For example, a large popcorn box that you buy at the movies can have more than 1,000 calories—even without butter. That's about two cheeseburgers worth of calories.

If you are obese, the first step toward reducing your knee pain, has to be in the area of reducing the weight you place on your knees. Mother Nature did not design the knee mechanism to take the excessive pounding of bone on bone. Denial can be a big problem for many people. Their weight problem catches up with them over a few years, and they refuse to confront the reality that they are now clinically obese. If your sore knees are the first signal from your body that you are overweight, act now to save your knees and improve your overall health.

Are you overweight and punishing your knees? Here's how to compute your own BMI

$$BMI = \frac{\text{Weight in pounds}}{\text{Height in inches squared}} \times 704.5$$

EXAMPLE: A six foot man weighing 180 pounds

$$BMI = \frac{180}{72 \text{ inches} \times 72 \text{ inches} = 5184} \times 704.5$$

$$24.46 = 0.0347222 \times 704.5$$

RANGES:
BMI less than 18.5 is UNDERWEIGHT
BMI 18.5 to 24.9 is IDEAL WEIGHT
BMI 25 to 29.9 is OVERWEIGHT
BMI 30 or above is OBESE

Are You Overweight?

Are you overweight? Here's a simple way to find out. Compute your Body Mass Index by taking your weight in pounds, divide that number by your height in inches squared, then multiple the result by 704.5. The U.S. Government says that if you have a BMI of twenty-five to twenty-nine, you are overweight. If your BMI is thirty or more, you are *obese.*

Diets run the gamut from sound to harmful, from sensible to faddish. Specific regimens are too numerous to count. Bookshelves are filled with them. If you are overweight, dieting may be necessary to reduce the unnecessary force you are placing on your knees. This is especially true for those suffering from arthritis. People who suffer from arthritis often find it difficult to lose weight because they find it painful to exercise away excess calories.

A typical lament is, "I am getting fat because I cannot exercise." It that is the case, try nonimpact sports like cycling or swimming. If these are impossible, you may have to focus more on your diet. Before embarking on a diet program, we strongly recommend that you meet with your personal doctor, or an internal medicine physician for specific diet recommendations that are best for you.

If you would rather do it yourself, go to www.guidelive.com, or many of the health Internet sites listed later on in this book, to find ways to eat healthy.

The Role of Food

Eating many of the foods, dietary supplements, vitamins, and minerals mentioned below may help relieve arthritis of the knee by providing the body with essential vitamins it needs to produce cartilage and collagen.

But there are some foods that seem to aggravate arthritis. Consumption of pepper, paprika, tobacco, cayenne, eggplant, and large amounts of tomatoes and potatoes is bad for arthritis because these foods contain alkaloids which prevent the repair of collagen and cartilage. Aspartame, the artificial sweetener, should also be avoided by arthritis sufferers because it causes inflammation and pain in the joints when consumed regularly or in large amounts.

Nooshin K. Darvish, a naturopathic physician in Seattle, recommends a diet rich in complex carbohydrates and fiber, which are found in whole grains, vegetables, and fruits. Also, she suggests that you reduce your fat intake. This type of diet will keep the excess weight off, which tends to put added stress on the joints. Darvish also recommends that you avoid caffeine and other stimulants because they deplete the body's supply of calcium, which is an important bone nutrient.

Dietary Supplements

In 1998, baseball player Mark McGwire was in the news for two reasons: First, he broke the all-time record for most home runs in a season. Second, he announced that he began taking Creatine, a sports supplement, at the beginning of the year. Over the past ten years, the sports supplement market has doubled in size to $1.3 billion, with women accounting for the majority of customers. Many women are looking for fat burners and other quick fixes.

One of the fastest growing areas is the new field dubbed nutriceuticals. Pills and powders that promise to help you lose weight and gain strength are marketed aggressively. Some are helpful, some are of no value whatsoever, and some can do harm. For example, there are cases of people who have had bad reactions to GBL (gamma butyrolactone), which is sometimes sold as a muscle builder. Part of the problem is that because physicians like to ignore the subject, trainers are playing that role by prescribing a variety of supplements to their clients, which can be dangerous.

We have tried to provide an overview here of some of the more well-known supplements. In many cases, this area is still so new that credible research is not yet available for many supplements.

Glucosamine and Chondroitin Sulfate

Nearly 40 million Americans, or one in seven people, have arthritis. For many, the arthritis causes pain in the knees and joints. Two very promising dietary supplements that have been shown to relieve arthritis are glucosamine and chondroitin sulfate.

Glucosomine and chondroitin sulfate are natural compounds that are taken from crab shells and cow cartilage. These compounds are also elements found naturally in your body. Your body makes glucosamine and chondroitin sulfate to build and protect the cartilage that cushions the ends of your bones. Glucosamine and chondroitin sulfate are often taken synthetically because the human diet lacks these naturally occurring elements.

Glucosamine is able to repair joints by providing the elements the joints need to repair the damage caused by injury or arthritis. The joint cartilage absorbs glucosamine and it helps to form cartilage by capping the ends of bones. Glucosamine also keeps the mechanisms that build and deteriorate cartilage balanced, thereby preventing unnecessary or untimely tissue loss.

Chondroitin keeps the enzymes in the knee from eating away at cartilage, and it helps other enzymes in moving the flow of nutrients to the cartilage in the knee. In test tube studies, chondroitin has been proven to stop certain enzymes from breaking down cartilage further.

Jane E. Brody, "Personal Health" columnist for the *New York Times*, says that European researchers have shown that glucosamine and chondroitin taken by mouth find their way to articular cartilage, and biopsies of some treated patients have shown structural improvements in damaged cartilage.

A study was conducted in the Department of Clinical Pharmacology in the Rotta Research Laboratory in Monza, Italy. They conducted three four to six week trials of glucosamine sulfate versus a placebo on 606 arthritis patients. The study found that glucosamine was effective in treating arthritis. Another study involving the elite Navy SEALs found that a combination of glucosamine (1,500 milligrams) and chondroitin (1,200 milligrams) relieved knee pain from extreme physical training.

Still another study, this one in the Rheumatology Division at the Case Western Reserve University School of Medicine in Cleveland, Ohio tested the effectiveness of glucosamine and chondroitin sulfate on hip and knee osteoarthritis. The study included trials over four weeks. Both glucosamine and chondroitin were tested with a placebo to determine their usefulness in treating osteoarthritis. All of the trials demonstrated that glucosamine and chondroitin were superior to the placebo in treating osteoarthritis of the knee and hip.

Notwithstanding the above, there is no scientific evidence at this time that proves these drugs rejuvenate joints damaged by arthritis. Unfortunately, there is no such drug at this time that will eradicate or reverse arthritis.

Because glucosamine and chondroitin are dietary supplements, the government does not require approval for these supplements to go on the market.

The only known side effects from glucosamine and chondroitin are nausea, diarrhea, constipation and heartburn. Researchers speculate that the supplements are not as harmful as traditional painkillers, which can cause stomach bleeding and liver or kidney damage when used long-term. If you have been using ibuprofen for knee pain and inflammation, you may want to give glucosamine and chondroitin a try. But be warned: A month's supply can cost $40 or more.

MSM

Methyl-sulfonyl-methane (MSM) is organic sulfur. It occurs naturally in the human body. MSM is also found in many foods. Milk contains the highest concentration of it. MSM also exists naturally in meat, vegetables, fruit, and seafood. The reason we do not get enough MSM is because so many of the foods we eat are processed. Washing and steaming also reduces MSM levels found in food. We take in less of it than our body requires because of this. As we grow older, our levels of MSM are also diminished.

Actor James Coburn is an outspoken advocate of MSM. For years, he suffered from rheumatoid arthritis, which became serious enough to prevent him from working. After taking MSM, however, Coburn was able to return to acting. He credits MSM for his comeback.

MSM is, for the most part, safe. A lethal dose of MSM in mice was more than twenty grams per kilogram of body weight. Thus, the probability of overdosing on MSM is extremely low.

Certain levels of MSM encourage healthy skin, nails, and hair. Higher levels of MSM can be used to help treat muscle soreness and cramps. The sulfur that occurs naturally in the body acts as an agent in many of the body's functions. One important function is the maintenance of connective tissue and the formation of collagen. Collagen is a protein which helps form bones. MSM increases the flow of harmful substances out of the cells and prevents pressure buildup in the cells, which causes inflammation in the joints. MSM is most widely used as an anti-inflammatory for joint and knee pain associated with arthritis.

Some studies have indicated that MSM improves joint flexibility, reduces stiffness and swelling, improves circulation, reduces pain associated with arthritis, reduces scar tissue, and breaks up the calcium deposits associated with arthritis. A study at Oregon Health Sciences University found that joint lesions in mice, which were similar to the lesions in rheumatoid arthritis reacted positively to MSM. They were given a 3 percent solution of MSM, and the researchers found that the mice suffered no degeneration of articular cartilage.

Shark Cartilage

Consider this amazing fact: The shark is a creature that has remained unchanged for 400 million years. It appears to be the only creature with a natural immunity to cancer and practically every disease known to man. Scientists believe that it is the shark's cartilage skeleton that provides this incredible immunity.

Shark cartilage is unique because it contains mucopolysaccharides, powerful anti-inflammatory molecules, in a concentration one thousand times greater than any other type of cartilage. It has also been found to contain small amounts of glucosamine and chondroitin.

Shark cartilage is now manufactured in capsules that can be taken as a dietary supplement to lessen the pain and stiffness in your knees. While it may not be 100 percent effective, it could help.

Shark cartilage is a nontoxic, natural supplement that contains calcium, phosphorous, and complex carbohydrates. The calcium and phosphorous is easily absorbed into the body, and the complex carbohydrates have been shown to reduce inflammation.

Using shark cartilage, Dr. Joseph Orcasity, a consultant at the University of Miami Medical School, treated a dozen elderly arthritis patients with severe knee pain. He reported that after taking shark cartilage for four weeks, most patients exhibited reduced pain and swelling and increased mobility.

Creatine

Creatine emerged on the scene in the late 1990s with many professional football players noting that they use the supplement to boost performance during intense exercise. Melvin Williams,

Ph.D., of Old Dominion University in Virginia, who is regarded by some as an expert in "ergogenic" or performance-boosting research in the United States, believes creatine works like caffeine and baking soda to buffer the lactic acid that builds up in muscles.

Gelatin

Research conducted at the Ball State Human Performance Laboratory showed that gelatin supplements have a positive effect on joint pain and stiffness in athletes. David Pearson, an associate professor of physical education, has been working with Nabisco to develop a gelatin supplement to promote healthy joints.

Ball State athletes with knee pain were recently tested. They included both male and female athletes participating in all sports. The post-evaluation showed that the gelatin supplements did indeed have a positive effect on knee pain.

Don't think that eating huge bowls of Jell-O will make your knees start feeling better. The gelatin supplement comes in a capsule form, which has a much greater concentration. The Food and Drug Administration has given the gelatin supplement a rating of GRAS (Generally Regarded as Safe).

Whey Protein/Glutamine

Protein smoothies and energy bars are everywhere these days, many with whey protein—a cheese by-product that is rich in the amino acid glutamine. It's believed that glutamine helps fuel white blood cells, which are key to the immune system. A 1996 British study, for example, followed marathon runners who took glutamine. They had a third fewer infections during the week after a race than those who did not take it.

Minerals

Several minerals have anti-inflammatory properties, and others act as antioxidants. According to Dr. Jason Theodosakis, who specializes in preventive medicine, minerals like boron, copper, silicon, manganese, and zinc are all important in treating osteoarthritis, and they aid your general health. Currently, research is being conducted to prove the usefulness of these minerals on arthritis. Minerals can be derived from many of the foods we eat, or they can be taken as a supplement.

Boron

Boron is used in calcium and bone metabolism, and it is an antioxidant and an anti-inflammatory. Dr. Theodosakis says that there is a correlation between the boron intake and osteoarthritis, which causes knee and joint pain. In areas of the body where osteoarthritis is high, there is less boron.

Normal joints have almost twice the level of boron than joints with osteoarthritis. Regardless of whether boron is, in fact, a proven cure for osteoarthritis, it does possess natural anti-inflammatory properties, which help the joint and tissue swelling associated with osteoarthritis. Boron can be found naturally in grapes, plums, dried fruit, nuts, grains, and leafy vegetables.

Calcium

The recommended dosage of calcium is 1,000 to 1,500 milligrams a day. The national average consumed is 750 milligrams a day. It is a proven fact that a lack of calcium contributes to osteoporosis. At the same time, it has not been proven that extra calcium will prevent osteoarthritis or joint pain. Because calcium is a natural antioxidant, it may help cleanse the joints of harmful toxins and by-products, which may cause cartilage degeneration. Calcium can be found in various dairy products, salmon, shrimp, whole grains, green leafy vegetables, almonds, broccoli, tofu, cabbage, asparagus, and oysters.

Copper

Copper is a mineral found in the enzymes that create bone

and collagen. Taking copper as a mineral supplement may help aid collagen formation in the joints of the knees. While there may not be a direct correlation between copper and the relief of arthritis, copper is an antioxidant, which can be taken to rid joints of toxins and by-products. Copper is found in nuts, mushrooms, barley, salmon, potatoes, legumes, shellfish, soybeans, and oatmeal.

Manganese

Like copper, manganese is part of many enzymes that form cartilage. Scientists have recognized a correlation between low levels of manganese and joint problems in animals. Because there is some evidence of a decline in the body's ability to use manganese as it increases in age, taking it as a supplement might aid in cartilage formation and help knee pain. You can get manganese from eating whole grains, peas, spinach, avocados, dried beans, egg yolks, pineapple, nuts, and blackberries.

Silicon

Silicon's function is to strengthen connective tissues that are made up of collagen. It is also important in forming bone and cartilage. People who have low bone density usually have very low levels of silicon. Silicon can be found in potatoes, cereal, apples, green vegetables, brown rice, and seafood. Obtaining silicon by eating these foods is a better way to consume this mineral, but it can also be taken in very small doses as a supplement.

Zinc

Zinc is a mineral that is known to greatly aid in wound healing. Like copper, zinc is also an important element that helps enzymes in the formation of cartilage and cartilage metabolism. Dr. Theodosakis says that several studies conducted on patients with both rheumatoid and psoriatic arthritis have shown that zinc supplements are beneficial when compared to the placebo in the reduction of joint pain and tenderness. Zinc is found in grains, nuts, red meat, potatoes, seafood, poultry, milk, eggs, soybeans, and mushrooms.

Vitamins and Their Effect on Our Bodies

Rheumatoid arthritis is a form of arthritis that causes extreme pain in the joints. Experts believe that rheumatoid arthritis is caused by an autoimmune disorder. This immune disorder affects the entire body by attacking the tissues. In rheumatoid arthritis, the immune disorder manifests itself in the joints. That is why people who have rheumatoid arthritis may suffer from knee pain. Vitamins contain many antioxidant properties and are used to help the immune system in flushing out toxins and cell by-products, which contribute to rapid cartilage breakdown.

Vitamin E

Vitamin E has been used for many purposes. It is taken frequently by those suffering from leg cramps, or knee pain related to arthritis or athletic injury. Vitamin E is a natural antioxidant that works to prevent the by-products of chemical-cell interaction, which cause cell damage. This works in treating arthritis, because it helps get rid of the calcium deposits around the joints, which are often associated with arthritis, and it stops the breakdown of cartilage. Vitamin E is found naturally in broccoli, peanut butter, asparagus, avocado, sunflower seed, and whole grain bread.

Vitamin C

Like vitamin E, vitamin C is a natural antioxidant, which has been used to help people with arthritis. Vitamins with the properties of synthetic antioxidants provide a safe way to relieve pain without the possible harmful side effects. Typically, your body needs more vitamin C than it gets from the foods you consume. Bioflavonoids are usually found in vitamin C tablets. These are plant chemicals containing antioxidant properties, which prevent the destruction of collagen caused by inflammation.

Vitamin C is found in many fruits like strawberries, oranges, cantaloupe, grapefruit, bananas, kiwi, and papaya. It is also found in parsley, tomatoes, spinach, cabbage, red pepper, and broccoli.

Vitamin D

Doctors have known for years that lack of vitamin D causes rickets and other bone problems. A 1996 study published by the journal *Annals of Internal Medicine* demonstrated that the lack of vitamin D also increases the onset of osteoarthritis. Vitamin D is made naturally by your body when it is exposed to the sun, and it is found in fortified milk, many seafood products, and cod liver oil.

Getting too much vitamin D can be toxic, so consult a doctor before ingesting a supplement along with your normal diet.

Vitamin B

Pantothenic acid has been shown to help arthritis pain and even prevent it. This acid exists as part of the vitamin B complex. Vitamin B helps the enzymes that are responsible for making collagen and preventing the rapid metabolism of cartilage. Vitamin B is found in broccoli and green leafy vegetables.

What about Alternative Medicine for Knee Problems?

Each year Americans spend an incredible amount of money on alternative medicine to treat a variety of pain complaints and ailments.

To put this in perspective, consider all the costs associated with hospitalizations each year in the United States. Amazingly, last year Americans spent about the same amount of money on alternative treatments. What makes this even more amazing is that because health insurance typically does not cover alternative treatments, patients generally pay for them out-of-pocket.

David Eisenberg, M.D., conducted a telephone survey which was published in the *Journal of the American Medical Association*. It demonstrated that alternative therapy use is growing. In 1997, the percentage of the U.S. population that sought alternative care increased from 33.8 percent (60 million people) to 42.1 percent (83 million people). Visits to alternative care providers in 1997 totaled 628,825,000. Visits to primary care physicians totaled only 385,919,000.

Over the last ten years there has been an explosion of interest in the new field of "nutraceuticals"—nutritional aids and dietary supplements that claim to make us healthier, happier, sleep better, more immune to cancer, etc.

Do alternative medicine solutions work? In some cases, some alternative medicines are worth exploring. In other cases, they are a complete waste of time. And in some other cases, they may make the situation worse.

As a general rule of thumb, we believe it is desirable to avoid surgery. But sometimes, a certain type of knee injury—such as a completely torn ligament, or bone fracture—may require surgery if you ever hope to regain mobility in that knee joint. In some cases, even delaying the surgery can cause further damage to the knee. Ask you knee doctor what would happen if you were to delay surgery. If waiting does not further damage the knee, you may want to wait a period of time to see if you can recover without surgery.

The American Medical Association's (AMA) spokesman, Jim Fox, says that the AMA encourages doctors to be aware of alternative therapies and to use them when appropriate.

Alternative medicine is loosely defined as a treatment that has not been strictly proven to aid an illness or injury, but it seems to aid the discomfort, pain, or symptoms from which one is suffering. It has been argued by many experts that these alternative medicine "cures" have a placebo effect on a patient. The patient believes the alternative cure is working, but really it is the patient's imagination that the pain is lessening.

Some of the treatments in this chapter date back thousands of years. While they may actually be valuable aids in healing, it is important to realize that they have not been strictly proven to cure what is ailing your knee.

It is also important to realize that if you use these alternative therapies indiscriminately, you could cause more damage to your knee and your overall health. Rather, alternative medicine should be used moderately as a supplement to proven therapy. If you do have troubling knee pain, it is a good idea to see a doctor in order to determine if the problem is serious. If you let the knee pain go undiagnosed, and you do not seek medical advice, the injury or discomfort could get worse.

Researching Alternative Medicine Solutions

The term "alternative medicine" is now dated. There is really nothing "alternative" anymore to some of the treatments consumers have made mainstream.

One of the problems with alternative medicine, however, is that traditional medical doctors are uninformed about it. That, in turn, forces the consumer to look elsewhere for information. But those who have information about alternative medicine are the alternative medicine providers themselves, so the information is likely to be biased in their favor.

So how can you find credible information about alternative medicine? The National Center for Complementary and Alternative Medicine (NCCAM) was established by a Congressional mandate in 1992. The center is part of the National Institutes of Health, which is part of the United States Department of Health and Human Services.

The center conducts biomedical research on alternative medicine. In 1993 they spent $2 million on alternative medicine research. That increased to $50 million in 1999. Instead of "alternative," the new buzzwords are "complementary" or "integrative" medicine, which more accurately reflects how these treatments are merging with mainstream medicine.

HMOs have responded to the strong consumer demand for complementary medical treatments, by including some, such as acupuncture, in their medical plans. A study conducted by Kaiser in 1998 found that 70 percent of adults wanted coverage for complementary treatments.

Some of the alternative remedies discussed have either been researched, or the research is currently in progress. For more guidance regarding research pertaining to alternative medicine and how to select an alternative medical practitioner see Chapter 10.

Herbs: a Natural Medicine

Rheumatoid arthritis and osteoarthritis are associated with the immune system. By boosting the immune system, herbs not only reduce inflammation, they also bolster the cell membranes. These membranes guard against diseases that produce painful inflammation. Among the herbs that reduce inflammation and contribute to immune system health are licorice, ginseng, cat's claw, and echinacea. Other herbs that contain anti-inflammatory properties are Chinese skullcap, devil's claw, curcumin, yucca, ginger, and witch hazel.

Cat's Claw & Devil's Claw

Cat's claw is a herb that comes from the Amazon and contains anti-inflammatory properties. Devil's claw is from the root of the plant Harpagophytum procumbens and it is used also to reduce pain and inflammation. A study conducted by the European Scientific Cooperation on Phytotherapy found that ten days of treatment with devil's claw provided significant pain relief.

Ginger

Ginger is a natural anti-inflammatory that may help knees. Unlike other synthetic anti-inflammatory medications, ginger will not irritate your stomach or cause long-term damage to your body.

Ginger has been documented as a proven anti-inflammatory in several studies. One reason for its amazing power as an anti-inflammatory is that it stimulates a change in the synthesis of the prostaglandin and leukotrines, which are hormone-like substances that reduce inflammation.

In her book, *Herbs for Health and Healing*, Kathi Keville, director of the American Herb Association asserts that ginger is highly effective in countering the symptoms of osteoarthritis and rheumatoid arthritis. She notes that a study regarding the use of ginger revealed that over 75 percent of the participants taking it found relief from these two conditions. Best of all, ginger has no harmful side effects.

Do not rely on cooked fresh ginger in your food to provide you with enough of the substance. Powdered ginger will be the most help. You can take two 500 mg capsules of ginger once or twice a day with food to reduce inflammation.

Nettles

Nettles are leaves from plants in Europe and Israel that are harvested and used for plant silica. Nettles are helpful in removing toxins from the body, including those cell by-products that interfere with cartilage formation. They have been used for quite some time for treating gout and other rheumatoid conditions. Nettles contain silica, potassium, sulfur, and vitamins A, C, and B. Because they are made up of these vitamins which have antioxidant and anti-inflammatory properties and minerals, they are useful in treating arthritis. You can buy this herb in capsule form over the counter.

Witch Hazel

More than one million gallons of witch hazel water are sold each year in the United States. Witch hazel was first used by Native Americans to heal cuts, bruises, insect bites, and aching muscles and joints. In the case of an ailing knee, witch hazel in the form of water or cream can be rubbed in to ease the soreness. It may also help diminish the appearance of bruises if your knee was visibly injured.

Alternative Treatments for Knee Pain

It is important to keep in mind that many of the following alternative treatments at best may relieve pain, and do little or nothing to change the structure of the knee. In that sense, these act as pain management alternatives. We do not endorse them as some may provide a little relief for some people, while others may note that they receive no benefit at all. With that caveat, here is an overview of alternative treatments for musculoskeletal pain complaints.

Acupressure

Acupressure is an ancient Chinese therapy. It is different from massage therapy and reflexology because it is administered by acupressurists who apply heavy pressure with their hands and feet to the points on the body that increase blood circulation and relieve pain. When pressure is applied to particular points on the body, muscles are relaxed and nerve fibers that cause pain are compressed. This compression may result in pain relief in the knee.

Acupressure is usually administered by a professional acupressure therapist. With some acupressure techniques, it can also be administered by yourself or by a partner at home.

Acupuncture

Acupuncture garnered some credibility in 1997 when the National Institutes of Health (NIH) endorsed it as a valid way to treat nausea and postoperative dental pain. The panel also agreed that acupuncture has value in treating conditions like headaches, lower-back pain, menstrual cramps, muscle pain, carpal tunnel syndrome, asthma, and some of the side effects caused by a stroke. The NIH Consensus Panel also found that acupuncture is an effective adjunct therapy for many conditions including muscle pain and osteoarthritis.

Knee pain is a condition that is commonly treated by acupuncture. According to the Food and Drug Administration report in 1993, up to 12 million visits to acupuncturists are made every year.

Acupuncture is an ancient Chinese form of alternative medicine. It has been in existence for over 3,000 years. It involves the insertion of hair-thin surgical needles into selected points on the body. The needles are stimulated by several methods which include pressure of the practitioner's hand, mild electric current, ultrasound, or wavelengths of light.

It is based on the belief that health is achieved through the harmonious balance between the opposing forces of yin (spirit) and yang (blood). Qi (pronounced "chi") is the attraction between the two forces. It flows to all parts of the body through channels called meridians. Meridians are pathways that run along the surface of the body and branch into the body's interior. Imbalance between those forces is believed to cause illness. When needles are inserted into the appropriate points along those meridians, balance is restored and health is regained.

Many doctors and researchers have speculated that acupuncture works not by achieving balance, but by stimulating pressure points and releasing endorphins. Whatever the case may be, acupuncture provides relief to many people suffering from pain.

The thought of needles may make you queasy, but this is

one alternative that has garnered much attention and credibility from the medical community. It is important if you seek this treatment that you rely on a licensed professional to administer it. Make sure the acupuncturist comes with a physician's referral, or they are certified by the National Commission for the Certification of Acupuncturists. For a list of certified acupuncturists in your area, call the American Association of Acupuncture and Oriental Medicine at (610) 266-1433.

Bee Venom

Bee venom therapy (BVT) has been around for many years, and it has been used to treat conditions like knee and joint pain. It was first pioneered by a Hungarian doctor in the 1930s. Lately, bee venom therapy has been used to treat multiple sclerosis. Patients suffering from this have used bee venom therapy to decrease leg and knee pain. Bee venom stresses a small part of the body's immune system. This trains the immune system to become stronger and build up tolerance to pain.

For example, if you are suffering from knee pain, bee venom therapy would be administered to the specific area of your knee that is causing you pain. Over time, the area that has been stressed by the BVT would grow stronger, and hopefully, the pain would diminish. It is important to remember that this therapy be administered only by a practitioner licensed in it.

Homeopathy

Homeopathy relies on the principle that a vegetable, animal, or mineral product that causes symptoms in a healthy person can cure those symptoms in an ill person when it is administered in appropriate doses. Homeopathy relies on stimulating the body's self-healing mechanisms by using highly diluted substances to trigger self-healing. The substances are usually administered in small doses and they come from minerals, animals, plants, conventional drugs, and synthetic chemicals.

Three basic principles of homeopathy are the principle

of similars, the minimum dose, and the holistic approach. The principle of similars takes into account the individualized symptoms of the disease. For example, rather than use an anti-inflammatory that would only help ease inflammation, homeopathic medicine would prescribe a certain herb or mineral that would not only act as an anti-inflammatory, but would also ease other symptoms of knee pain like a dull ache. The law of minimum dose relies on the introduction of a remedy in very small amounts. Then, the patient is monitored to determine if the remedy is working or if more needs to be administered.

The holistic approach of homeopathy mandates that when the patient is treated with the remedy, his or her physical, emotional, and psychological reactions are given equal attention. For example, if the patient has knee pain, but also has other symptoms like fatigue, then the ideal homeopathic remedy would not only reduce the knee pain and inflammation, but would also boost energy level.

Homeopathic drugs must meet Federal Drug Administration (FDA) standards of strength, quality, and purity. They must also comply with labeling and manufacturing requirements. However, the FDA does not require laboratory testing to determine the identity and strength of each active ingredient. Most physicians regard homeopathic treatment with some skepticism. However, there are some that practice it along with conventional medicine.

Jennifer Jacobs, M.D., a family practice physician in Washington state, specializes in homeopathic medicine. She is also sits on the National Institute of Health's Office of Alternative Medicine advisory committee. Dr. Jacobs uses homeopathy to help patients with chronic illnesses like arthritis and allergies that do not seem to respond to traditional treatments. Jacobs says that the traditional medicines may just mask the symptoms rather than actually heal them. She warns that nothing in medicine, either conventional or alternative, is absolute.

Hydrotherapy

Hydrotherapy came to the United States from Germany. Research has shown that aerated baths or spas have had positive effects on the body. Spas and whirlpools have been used as therapy to improve circulation and relieve chronic pain from the back and joints. Hydrotherapy relies on cold, warm, or hot water depending on the treatment. The use of cold water reduces inflammation, but the use of cold and warm water together can improve circulation.

Many doctors recommend whirlpool baths which help relieve arthritic joint pain, including knee pain. For inflammation, cold packs are sometimes used on the appropriate area. Dr. Nooshin K. Darvish recommends that patients apply moist heat to the knee for three minutes, alternating with one minute of moist cold. This hydrotherapy of placing hot and cold compresses on the knee will bring relief while stimulating circulation. Dr. Darvish says that by improving the circulation, the herbs taken by mouth for knee pain will be drawn to the affected area.

Liniments

Liniments have been used for centuries on sore muscles and joints. They do not repair torn ligaments or menisci, but can reduce soreness and stiffness induced by exercise. Ben Gay and Atomic Balm are liniments, which are available in most drugstores. They are believed to work by being "counter irritants," bringing a sense of warmth and tingling to a knee joint stiffened by overuse or injury. Once again, they do not cure the injury or disease, but render the symptoms less troublesome. They are typically used by trainers to get their hurting but not seriously injured players back on the field.

Magnetic Therapy

Most physicians are skeptical and advise patients to avoid magnets. Unfortunately, Americans aren't buying that. They're

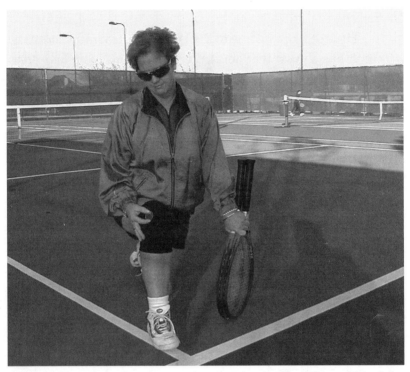

Laura Saurez, a former touring tennis pro who competed against Navratilova and Evert in her competitive days in the 1970s, now struggles with nagging knee pain from damaged cartilage. She copes by using a knee brace that holds a tiny circular magnet in place against the side of her knee. The magnet, shown outside the brace, slips inside the fabric brace. "I find that when I use the magnet, there isn't as much swelling or pain after tennis. Also, it doesn't limit my movement. It has definitely allowed me to continue to play tennis."

buying magnets—an estimated $200 million worth in 1998 alone. While traditional allopathic physicians wince at such statistics, the reality is that word of mouth is selling magnets for foot, back, leg, elbow, and other problems.

Magnets are used to treat many aches and pains. Advocates of magnetic therapy argue that magnetic flow assists in moving the blood through vessels. Normally, blood flows through veins and arteries. This allows for the exchange of fluids and nutrients. Sometimes knee pain results from poor circulation due to inadequate circulation of these nutrients through capillary walls. Magnets aid in moving the blood through the vessels to increase circulation and blood flow, which increases oxygen. This decreases inflammation and can limit your knee pain.

Magnets are marketed by many companies. Most of them offer their products over the Internet. Magnets can come in the form of knee braces, wrist bands and even mattress pads. Magnet therapy has received endorsements form professional athletes like Dan Marino of the Miami Dolphins, Bill Romanowski of the Denver Broncos, and pro golfer Chi Chi Rodriguez.

Like most M.D.s, Carlos Vallbona, M.D., a rehabilitation specialist at the Baylor College of Medicine in Houston, was critical of magnets. So he put together a thoughtfully crafted study. He had a magnet manufacturer make two different sets of magnets, identical in appearance, except one set had no magnetic power. The identity of each set was closely guarded with a secret code. Neither patients nor researchers knew which were the real magnets. He found that 76 percent reported that when the magnets were worn for forty-five minutes, their pain was significantly decreased compared to only 19 percent of the placebo patients with the nonfunctional magnets. He was stunned by the results, and is planning additional studies.

Other notable institutions are also claiming positive findings about magnets. New York Medical College and Vanderbilt University in Tennessee have both produced research favorable to magnets. Vanderbilt operates a clinic devoted to non-surgical treatment of chronic pain. Robert Holcomb, M.D., Ph.D., from the Neurology Department at Vanderbilt believes that magnetic energy alters the chemical interactions in nerve fibers that are responsible for pain impulses, which in turn interrupts the pain signal before it reaches the brain. This mechanism is similar to electrical nerve stimulation, which has been used in orthopedics for more than a decade.

While more research is sure to come in the next few years, the bottom line on magnet research can be summed up as follows: Some people find dramatic relief, some mild relief, and a good number of people find no relief whatsoever. Other areas that need more exploration include how often to apply magnets and the power of magnetic force needed. One thing to consider: Some magnet manufacturers boast that their magnets are different and better than another, and that might not be true. Researchers recommend magnets with a power of 500 to 1,000 gauss. One benefit of the popularity of magnets is that the prices are dropping. Even discount chains now offer generic magnets at a low price.

Secondly, magnets really do no harm—unless you place one near a pacemaker or other implanted medical device, which could affect its operation.

Remember, though, even if magnets help to relieve your pain, they can't cure the condition that is causing it. In this sense, they may at best be acting as a mild painkiller.

Massage Therapy

Pain caused by arthritis or an athletic injury can be soothed by massage therapy. Rather than massaging specific parts of the hands and feet, like reflexology, massage therapy is applied directly to the area that is afflicted.

In sports, many times massage is used not only to treat pain, but to prevent it. Muscles are massaged to warm them up to prevent strain before workouts or athletic events. The muscles can also be massaged after a workout to bring blood and oxygen into the muscles to flush out metabolic waste and increase circulation to the muscles to bring them the nutrients they need to heal after strenuous activity.

Likewise, arthritic joints and the muscles around the joints can be massaged to increase circulation. This brings the muscles and joints the nutrients they need to heal and to reduce inflammation. Another bonus of massage therapy is that it can break up adhesions and scar tissue in injured ligaments and muscles.

Relieving soreness or the "knot" in the over-used muscle is the task of the masseuse. Massage is commonly used in track and field, as well as cycling. Consider the Tour de France, the most prominent bike race in the world. Cycling teams from across the world routinely employ a masseuse dedicated to loosening the thigh muscles taxed by 100-mile days on a bike.

Reflexology

Reflexology was first practiced by the early Egyptians. It involves the massage of the hands and feet to stimulate a certain part of the body. For example, when the big toes are treated, there is a related effect on the head. If you are congested, a reflexologist would rub your big toe. Treating the whole foot would have an effect on the whole body. To relieve knee pain, a reflexologist would rub a corresponding area on the hands and feet to make the pain or discomfort better.

You or a partner can massage the appropriate area on the hand or foot to relieve knee pain. On the right foot, locate your arch. Across from the arch on the outside of the foot there is a triangular area, where the apex is even with the ankle bone, just south toward your toes, that can be massaged to help relieve knee pain. You can also massage the triangular, fleshy area on the outside edge of the right hand, just above the wrist to relieve knee and elbow pain.

Yoga, Zen, and Tai Chi

Many individuals have turned toward remedies which originated in the orient. Yoga, Zen, and Tai Chi are often touted as having some benefit.

Yoga has been popular as a disciplined means of increasing flexibility. Whether you are young or old, we recommend stretching limbs that have become tight through inactivity or sore from aggressive participation in sports. By increasing flexibility, you also decrease the risk of future injury from straining a tight, inflexible muscle, ligament, or tendon.

Zen, on the other hand, appears to have more benefit in the area of shaping mental state. The ability to concentrate, the will to strenuously train, or compete, or the composure to follow a strict and lengthy rehab program may be enhanced by the focus achieved through Zen. In our frenetically paced world, all of us need focus and discipline.

Tai Chi is a form of exercise and a stress management tool. If one were to observe a classroom of Tai Chi participants, they would look as if they were moving in slow motion. Tai Chi involves slow, methodical, and rhythmic movements of the arms and legs. While it appears easy, it is not, and can provide a strenuous but relaxing workout. Like Yoga and Zen, a side benefit of Tai Chi is that it works to improves one's perspective on life. In this sense, advocates argue that it has significant stress management benefits as well. For a knee pain sufferer, some of the leg movements may be difficult as they place body weight on the knee in certain positions.

A Final Note about Sports Supplements

If you have a question about sports supplements, go to the U.S. Food & Drug Administration's Internet site at www.fda.gov where you will find an overview of problem supplements. Click on the Food section, then Dietary Supplements. More information is also available at The Gatorade Sports Science Institute site at www.gssiweb.com, Nutrition Science News at www.nutritionsciencenews.com, and the Internet Society for Sports Science at www.sportsci.org. These sites cover a wide range of supplements and their side effects.

Chapter 6

Exercises To Relieve Knee Pain, Strengthen the Knee, and Get You Moving Again

For someone suffering knee pain the mere thought of exercise can be painful.

For most knee problems specific exercises help rehabilitate injured tissues, strengthen weak muscles, and improve flexibility and range of motion.

Doing the exercises in this chapter may also reduce the risk of future injury. A 1998 study by the Alfred I. DuPont Institute revealed that athletes who stretched their thigh muscles, reduced the incidence of knee pain. The researchers studied 149 athletes who had no previous knee pain or knee injury. The athletes were instructed to do flexibility exercises at morning and night, and before and after participating in their sport. Subsequent knee pain symptoms during sports were reduced in 129 of the cases.

This chapter can benefit most people suffering from routine knee problems, especially those who have just noticed some knee symptoms coming on over a period of time. In this book, all the various exercises related to the knee are presented in Chapter 6 and Chapter 9.

The exercises are separated according to the following rationale: Those people who are in pain currently from knee problems should start with the exercises in this chapter. If you make progress and start to get moving again on your own, fantastic. Continue on to the exercises in Chapter 9. If you don't and your knee problem persists, then it may be time for you to explore the assistance of a good knee specialist, and follow his or her recommendations.

If you need to go down the surgery path, then you must read Chapter 8, which provides guidance on how to select the best knee specialist. You must take responsibility for the choices you make when you enter the health care system. If you choose the wrong doctor, or a doctor who does not have sufficient experience in your type of knee surgery, beware. You may be increasing your risk of more problems down the road. Just as you would research the purchase of your next car, spend an equal amount of time researching the doctor who will affect how mobile you may be throughout the rest of your life. You can always sell a car that turns out to be a lemon. You can't replace your knees.

Those people dealing with traumatic injury, such as a fall that has torn a ligament or banged the kneecap, should *not* embark on any knee exercise program until they have been examined by a physician. A fall on the knee or a blow to it could have caused a bone fracture, and exercise could worsen the situation. But for many people with knee pain that comes on gradually, trying some of the exercises in this chapter can increase mobility. Those people who suffer from arthritis, for example, may benefit greatly from the easy exercises in Chapter 6 and tougher exercises in Chapter 9. Unfortunately, arthritis is a degenerative condition that doesn't much lend itself to surgical repair. On the positive side, however, there is growing scientific research that exercise and motion in an arthritic joint can relieve some arthritis pain symptoms and increase range of motion in the joint.

Before You Get Started on Your Knee Exercises

For those people with knee pain, the goal of the exercises in this chapter is to strengthen the knee muscles outside the "pain zone." Many people with knee problems can still move the knee joint through a certain range of motion without pain, or with only mild discomfort. You begin your exercise program by working in those zones, which are relatively comfortable, and through these exercises, expand those zones to a wider range.

If you have knee pain, remember the purpose of these exercises is to strengthen the knee and leg muscles *outside* those zones that cause pain. Do not force your knee to perform motions in a zone that generates acute pain. For instance, certain motions should be avoided by those people with anterior knee pain, that is, pain around the front of the knee. Anterior knee pain can be caused by irritation under the kneecap or patellar tendinitis. Your patellar tendons operate much like rubber bands that go from the bottom of the front of your thigh, through the kneecap, to the front of the shin. When these tendons become irritated or sore, extending or straightening the leg can be painful. Consequently, people with this type of anterior knee pain should avoid extension exercises that force the leg to straighten, especially if they cause pain.

Another group that should avoid extension exercises are those people who have just undergone surgery to replace their torn anterior cruciate ligament, where the surgeon harvested part of the patellar tendon to act as the new ACL. Extension exercises are not recommended for this population, as the patellar tendon is already weakened from the surgery and needs time to heal. As a general rule of thumb, if you had any type of knee surgery, follow your own knee doctor's exercise program.

Think you'd rather have surgery than do any of these knee exercises? Consider this: Even those people who may ultimately need knee surgery, can benefit from simple exercises and movements outside the pain zone. That's because after surgery your knee will be weakened and you must then begin the tedious and painful journey back through physical therapy and rehabilitation, i.e., exercise. The more you are able to strengthen supporting leg muscles and hip flexors before surgery, the easier your rehab will be after surgery.

How Chapter 6 and Chapter 9 Exercises Differ

The exercises in Chapter 6 are relatively easy on the knee joint. They are good for someone attempting motion with simple knee pain, or during the recovery process after surgery. For example, if you have surgery, chances are your knee doctor will have you doing some of the exercises in this chapter after your surgery to get your knee joint moving again.

If you are able to do most of the exercises in Chapter 6, then you can proceed to some of the tougher exercises in Chapter 9. In many cases, the exercises in Chapter 9 use the weight of your body on the knee joint. This is one of the reasons you should never start your knee exercise program with the exercises shown in Chapter 9. If you begin a squat movement, for example, and your knee buckles under your body weight, you could damage weakened ligaments or further hurt yourself.

In addition to placing more weight demand on the knee, the exercises in Chapter 9 are really set up to simulate certain movements inherent in various sports. Skiing, for example, requires the knee to play the role of shock absorber as you maneuver down a mountain over moguls. Consequently, you will find jumping exercises that simulate the impact that your knee will face out on the slope.

When doing any of the exercises with a sore knee, we recommend doing the same movement, even the simple exercises, with the healthy knee as well. As the exercises become more challenging, you will strengthen the healthy knee which will help support the body as it moves back into activity.

Lastly, in this book we emphasize the use of a Sportcord, which enables you to create resistance without having to go to the gym or purchase expensive weight machines. The Steadman-Hawkins Clinic in Vail, Colorado recommends the use of a Sportcord for their celebrity athletes as they recover from shoulder and knee injuries. In the back of the book, you will find phone and Internet ordering information, as well as a coupon for a discount off the purchase price.

So let's get started slowly with the simple knee exercises shown in this chapter. Hopefully, they'll get your knee moving well enough that you don't have to go down the surgical path covered in Chapters 7 and 8. Anytime you can safely avoid or delay surgery, you're moving in the right direction.

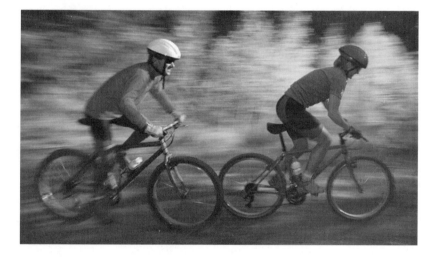

Simple Knee Extension

Overview: This is a subtle and easy exercise that encourages full extension of the leg. This can be done as a warm-up for the straight leg raises that come next. Sit as shown with both legs straight. Try to lower the back of your knee so it touches the floor. Hold for five seconds then relax. Repeat twenty times. An alternative would be to place a towel under the back of the ankle to encourage full extension.

Straight-Leg raise

Overview: You should make sure the leg is locked straight and there is no flexion or extension of the knee joint. This exercise works the hip flexor muscles and the upper quadriceps muscle in the upper thigh area. How to do it: There are several ways to do this exercise depending on how difficult it seems to you. The easiest starting position may be to start with a rolled-up towel supporting the back of your knee. If you use the towel, make sure your leg does not bend and extend. If you need more resistance, you could also add an ankle weight. The goal is to raise the leg in a straightened position about one foot off the floor. Keep your toe up and back. Hold for ten seconds, and go back to the starting position. As seen in fig. 2, it can also be done without the towel. Repeat ten times.

Knee Flexion Exercise

Overview: This is another simple range of motion exercise for the knee that uses the weight of the leg for resistance. This exercise helps increase flexibility as well as strengthens the hamstrings.

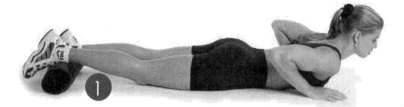

How to do it: Start by lying on your stomach, with your upper body supported by your elbows. Place one foot on a rolled up towel and slowly raise it upward six inches off the towel, hold for five seconds, then slowly return to horizontal. Repeat twenty times, and then switch legs.

Full Flexion

Overview: This exercise flexes the knee to ninety degrees.

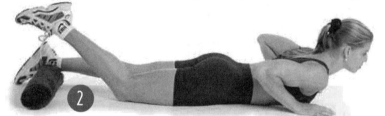

How to do it: Raise the foot up and back to ninety degrees, hold for five seconds, then return to start. Repeat twenty times.

Horizontal Straight-Leg Raise with Chair

Overview: This exercise strengthens the upper leg muscles that support the knee joint. Because this exercise doesn't require any painful bending of the knee, it can be done while recovering from a knee injury. *How to do it:* Use two chairs or a chair across from a sofa. While seated, extend your leg so that it rests on the other chair. Slowly raise the leg no more than twelve inches, keeping it straight during the motion. Hold for ten seconds, then return to starting position. Repeat ten times for each leg.

Straight-Leg Lift Exercise

Overview: This exercise strengthens supporting muscles in the leg, while not requiring any movement in the knee joint area.

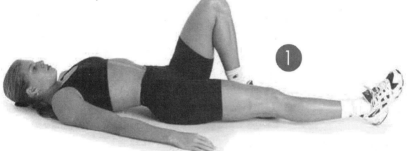

How to do it: Start by lying on your back with your left leg bent upward. Keep your right leg completely extended straight out. Slowly raise your right leg to about a forty-five degree angle, keeping the leg locked straight. Hold for five seconds and then slowly lower to the flat, resting position. It is not necessary to take the leg straight up to ninety degrees, as the most difficult range of motion is the first two feet off the ground. Repeat twenty times. Switch to the left leg.

Toe Rotation

Overview: This exercise combines a straight leg raise with rotation of the leg, which works the lower quadriceps muscle. How to do it: Raise the leg in a straightened position about one foot off the ground. Then with your toe up, rotate the foot to the left and then back to the

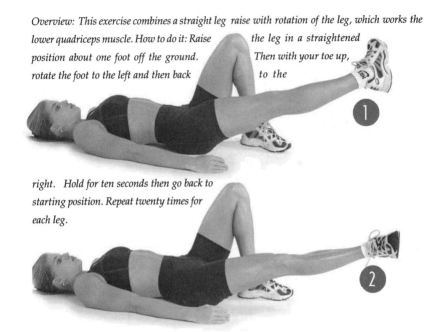

right. Hold for ten seconds then go back to starting position. Repeat twenty times for each leg.

Leg ADduction

Overview: "ADduction" is an exercise where the movement is inward, "ABduction" is where the movement is outward. How to do it: As shown, start with one foot above the chair, and one below resting on the ground.

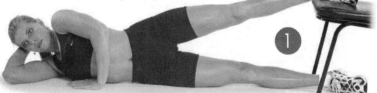

Raise the straightened leg upward against the bottom of the chair.
Hold for ten seconds and then return the leg to the floor. Repeat ten times, then switch legs.

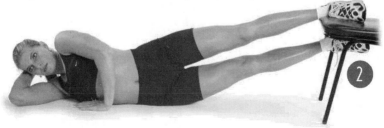

Leg Raise ABduction Exercise

Overview: Rather than focusing on the knee joint itself, the purpose of this exercise is to strengthen the supporting muscles of the upper leg, including the outer thigh area. How to do it: Start by lying on your side with your lower leg bent behind you, as shown, for balance. Slowly raise your

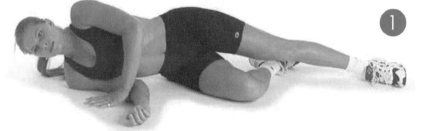

upper leg while keeping it straight. Hold for five seconds, then slowly lower back to the starting position. Do twenty repetitions, repeat with the other leg.

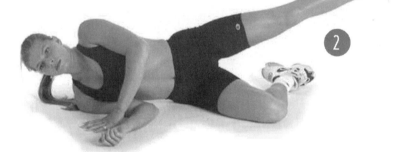

Knee Slide

Overview: This is a simple stretch for the upper leg, also involving some flexion in the knee area without resistance. How to do it: Start with your right leg bent as shown, foot flat on the ground. Slowly slide your toe backward until the knee is fully bent. Hold for five seconds, then slide the foot back to the starting position. Repeat ten times and then switch legs.

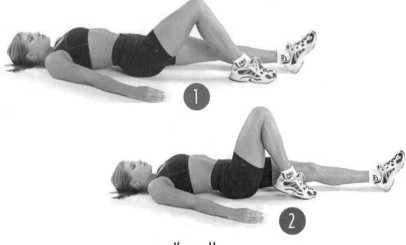

Knee-Up

Overview: This is a simple stretching exercise for the quadriceps and knee. How to do it: Start with both legs straight, as shown. Raise your left leg until the upper thigh is perpendicular to the ground. There is no need to go farther than a ninety degree angle. Hold for five seconds, and then return to starting position. Repeat ten times, and then switch legs.

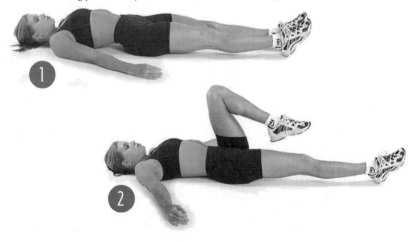

"Unweighted Exercises"
Leg Cycle Exercise

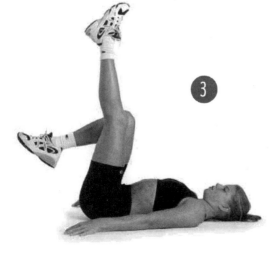

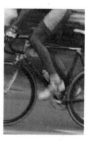

Overview: A healthy knee joint has freedom of movement. Sometimes walking, running, or cycling present too much of a load-bearing demand on a painful knee. The purpose of this exercise is to encourage movement in the knee but without the weight or resistance that may cause discomfort.

How to do it: Start by lying on your back with both legs upward. Extend both your arms out at your sides for balance. Begin a cycling motion with your feet in the air. Try to increase the range of motion in the knee joint area, so the flexion in each leg goes from almost straight and extended to bent at a ninety degree angle.

Straight-Leg Piriformis Stretch

Overview: The piriformis is a muscle that runs through the buttock area into the back of the thigh. It is common for a piriformis muscle to tighten and shorten from sitting. In fact, the common position of driving where the knees are apart, further encourages the piriformis to shorten and then strain itself with subsequent activity. Many times, the symptoms of lower back pain can be relieved with this stretch as well. The benefit for the knee area is that this stretch is beneficial to the upper leg which supports the knee area. How to do it: Lie on your back as shown. Raise your left leg and bring it across your body, trying to make it touch the ground by your right hand. Keep both your shoulders flat to the ground. *Hold for twenty seconds, then return to starting position and repeat for the other leg. Do ten repetitions with each leg.*

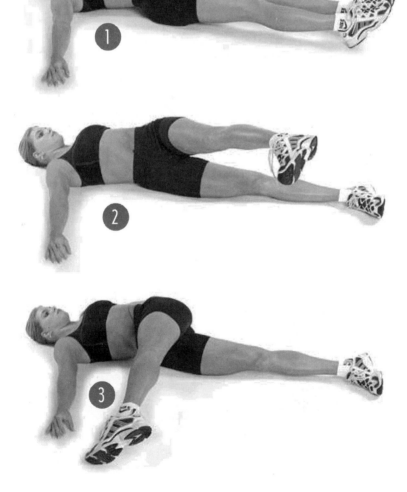

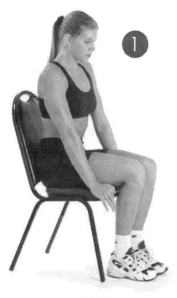

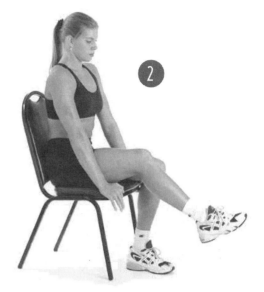

Knee Full Extension Exercise

Overview: This is a simple range of motion exercise for the knee that just uses the weight of the leg for resistance. As simple as this exercise looks, it can be very difficult when recovering from surgery. This exercise should not be done when you are recovering from ACL repair surgery and when the patellar tendon was used to replace the torn ACL.

How to do it: Start by sitting in a chair that is high enough so that the knee can bend to a ninety degree angle. Slowly raise the leg until it is horizontal. Hold for five seconds, and slowly let it return to the ground. Repeat with other leg. Do twenty repetitions, if able.

Knee Stretch

Overview: This knee stretch should not be done on a sore knee where you are not sure of the underlying problem. How to do it: Start with your right leg slightly bent as shown, and with your left leg crossed over the other. Grab the right leg at the back of the thigh and pull toward the chest until the right leg is straight up, but no farther. Hold for five seconds, then return to starting position. Switch legs and repeat. Do ten repetitions with each leg. Discontinue if the exercise causes more pain to your sore knee.

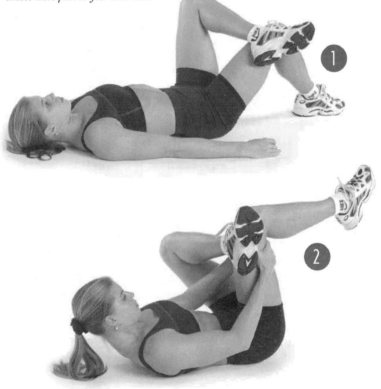

Double Knee To Chest

Overview: This is a great stretch for the legs and lower back. How to do it: Start on your back with your legs outstretched. Bring both knees up together and place your hands below the knee area on the top of the shin. An alternative place for your hands is the back of the thighs. Slowly bring your knees toward your chest, hold for ten seconds, then go back to starting position.

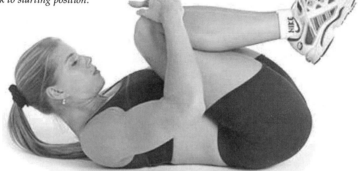

Ankle Stretch

Overview: Supporting muscles in the leg can either assist your knee, or make it do extra duty in stabilizing the weight of our upper bodies as you walk. This exercise strengthens the lower leg so it can support a weak knee. How to do it: Place one end of a Sportcord over your right foot at the instep (not the tip of the shoe). Extend your right leg and pull up the Sportcord until you have the desired resistance and difficulty. Extend your right toe downward, as if you are pressing on the gas pedal in your car. Hold extended for five seconds, and then repeat twenty times. Switch legs and start from the beginning.

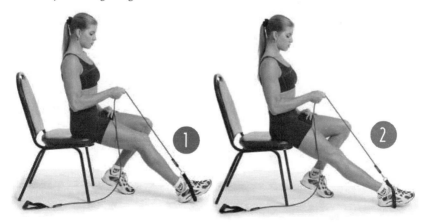

Front Step-Up

Overview: This exercise requires the knee to straighten and raise the body weight. How to do it: Use a platform or several large books to make a six to eight-inch step. Stand in front of the step and with your right leg, step up. Avoid locking your leg, and try to hold the position for three seconds before stepping back down. Switch legs and repeat. Do ten repititions with each leg.

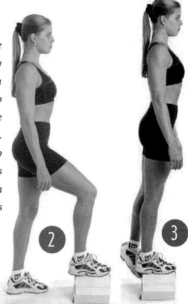

Unweighted Flexion

Overview: This is a simple flexion exercise for the knee. How to do it: Stand behind a chair using the back of the chair for balance. Flex your left leg up to about a ninety degree angle, hold for ten seconds, then go back to starting position. Switch legs, and do ten repetitions with each leg.

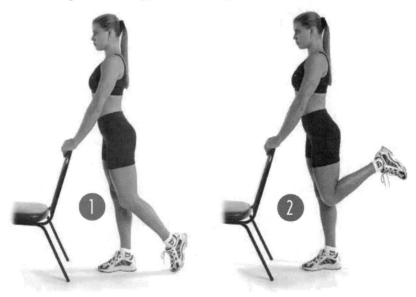

Side Steps

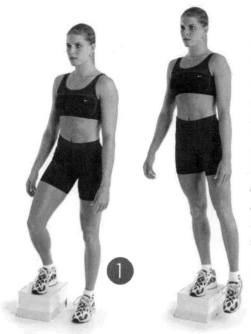

Overview: This exercise requires the knee to straighten and raise the body weight from a sideways step-up position. How to do it: Use a platform or several large books to make a six-to-eight-inch step. Stand next to the step and using your right leg, step up. Avoid locking your leg, and try to hold the position for three seconds before stepping back down. Switch legs and repeat. Do ten repetitions with each leg.

Flexion with Weights

Overview: This exercise is a variation of the exercise on the previous page, only with an ankle weight to add resistance. How to do it: Add an ankle weight and flex the ankle upward to a ninety degree angle. Hold for five seconds. Repeat the exercise ten times, then switch legs.

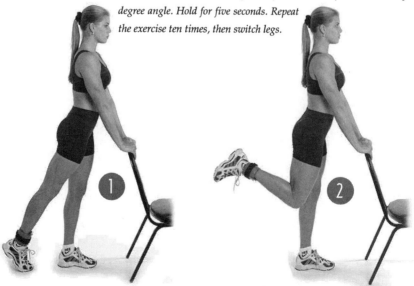

Single Hamstring Stretch

Overview: The hamstrings, which run up the back of the thigh, are crucial to stabilizing the weight of the upper body. Hamstrings are also prone to strain. This exercise improves the flexibility and strength of the hamstring.

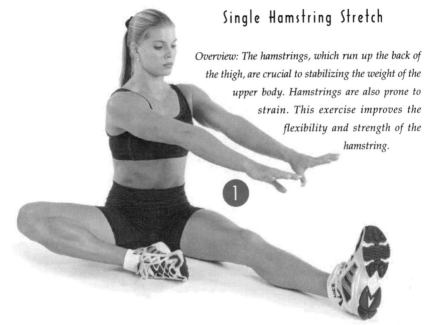

How to do it: Sit on the floor with your left leg outstretched and your right leg bent as shown. With both hands extended, reach out toward your toes of the left foot. Don't bounce, just stretch slowly. Try to hold the stretch for ten seconds, then go back to the starting position. Do ten repetitions before switching legs.

Double Hamstring Stretch

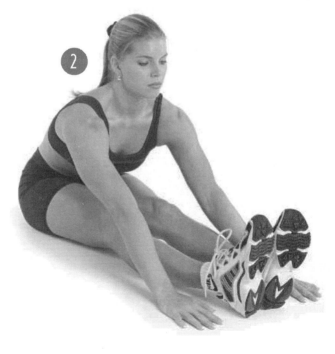

Overview: One of the natural side effects of our sedentary lifestyle is that too much sitting naturally shortens our hamstrings. This is another variation of the hamstring stretch, in which both hamstrings are stretched simultaneously. This position can be better if bending the knee is uncomfortable for your sore knee. How to do it: Start with both legs extended as shown. Extend your hands down toward your ankles, trying to keep your palms pressed flat throughout the movement. Hold the stretch for ten seconds, and repeat twenty times.

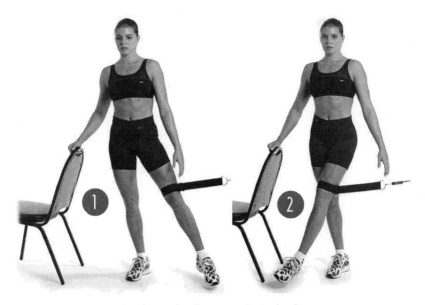

Thigh ADduction and ABduction

Overview: This exercise uses the resistance of a Sportcord to strengthen the inner thigh (see ADduction above) and outer thigh (see ABduction below). How to do the above exercise: Anchor one end of the Sportcord to a doorknob on a closed door. Place the belt two inches above the knee, not on the knee. Holding the back of a chair as shown, swing the left leg inward and across. Repeat ten times, and then   switch legs. Below: Place the Sportcord belt on the   thigh farthest from the doorknob.   Swing out and away from the doorknob.

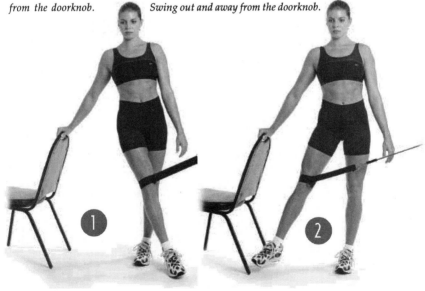

Lunges

Overview: This is an advanced exercise that works the entire knee area. But because this exercise places your body weight on a single knee you may want to be cautious. An alternative position would be to use the back of a chair as a crutch. Also, those with anterior knee pain, like patellar tendinitis, quadriceps tendinitis, or those recovering from ACL repair, in which the patellar tendon was used, should avoid this exercise initially. How to do it: Start with right leg extended as shown. Slowly and carefully, go forward and down until the left knee touches the ground. Hold the stretch for five seconds, and go back to starting position, using a small recovery step on the way back. Switch legs and repeat. Do ten repetitions with each leg.

Aerobic Exercise and Being Overweight

With the exception of some of the advanced ski exercises in Chapter 9, the knee exercise program is not to replace your aerobic exercise program, which is also essential. Body weight is a key factor in knee pain. This is problematic for people who find themselves overweight and with knee pain. That's because to lose weight, you need to exercise to speed up your metabolism. But most aerobic exercises, like running, biking, aerobic classes, jazzercise, etc., all involve the knees. Consequently, a knee pain sufferer who is overweight may feel they are stuck. They can't exercise, so weight can pile on, and more weight places more pressure on sore knees.

There is a way out. A stationary bike is a great aerobic exercise that doesn't put too much of a load on the knee joint. But it does require a full range of motion. If that's a problem, most gyms have a machine that looks like a stationary bike, only the pedals are for the hands and arms. This machine gets the heart rate up just like a stationary bike, only the legs do nothing. Another alternative is to swim. There is no impact, and even if you choose to kick, the range of motion is slight.

There is no shortage of books and diet plans geared toward losing weight, so we do not cover that in this book. Consult your personal doctor for his or her advice on how to alter your diet to lose weight. Once your weight is down, your knee health will likely improve. Another point to keep in mind if your knee pain has you feeling down and out: Exercise has been proven to be great medicine for depression. Research published in *Professional Psychology: Research and Practice* noted that researchers in fourteen separate depression studies found exercise to be beneficial. Depression was lessened even in patients who only ran or walked twenty minutes three times a week for five weeks. The researchers also noted that exercise was beneficial in relieving chronic pain, as well.

Chapter 7

When Surgery Must Be Considered

When the knee is injured badly or when the joint is destroyed by arthritis, recovery will require a knee surgeon. Of all those people sitting in the doctor's waiting room for knee trauma, 20 percent, or one in five people, will need surgery. This chapter may motivate you to do those exercises to strengthen your knees, and to use a little more caution the next time you choose to hit the moguled double diamond or lunge for a drop volley or rebound.

In this chapter we discuss which knee injuries require surgery and how it is done. Many patients these days want to see exactly how a procedure works. We felt that by picturing knee surgery, we could provide that kind of detailed information. Consequently, we walk the reader through two common knee surgeries. Some readers will find such photographs fascinating; others may find them too explicit and unsettling. We believe that when it comes to health care, you cannot have too much information. With that said, let's step into the operating room.

Within the surgical suite, there are two classes of people: those who are in contact with the "sterile field" and those who assist. The "sterile field" includes the patient and any attached surgical tables with instruments. Those within the sterile field, not only wear scrubs, but wear a sterile surgical gown and gloves. They do not come into contact with those outside the sterile field.

And those outside the sterile field stay clear of even the draping that may extend off a table that holds the surgical instruments.

Sound impressive? When a total knee replacement is being performed the sterile approach is racheted up several notches. Even air flow within the room is controlled. The surgeons wear space suits, which further protect the surgical field from infection. Infection within a total joint can be significant and debilitating. Consequently, expertise and technological sophistication are required not just of the surgeon, but the entire team. Now that you understand sterile fields, let's catch up with the ACL replacement that is taking place in OR one and total knee replacement in OR two.

Repair of the Torn Anterior Cruciate Ligament

The photos that follow take you through the surgery that is done to repair a fully torn ACL. ACL repair is a procedure that has been around for decades, but over approximately the last ten years it has been done through tiny holes rather than a major incision in the knee.

There are two main differences in how the ACL may be repaired, based on where the new ligament is harvested. Some doctors remove a strand of the patellar tendon to make a new ACL, while others favor harvesting part of the hamstring for the job. While the hamstring method is far more popular and common today among orthopedic surgeons, there are strong advocates for the patellar tendon method. Dr. Garrett performs virtually all ACL repairs by harvesting two strands from the hamstring in the back of the thigh. This method has proven successful for amateur and professional athletes. While initially the strength of the hamstring is compromised, over time the fibers grow together to return the hamstring back to its original strength. On the other hand, the Steadman-Hawkins Clinic in Vail, Colorado has for years been the first choice for injured celebrity athletes. Dr. Hawkins, who specializes in shoulders, and Dr. Steadman, who excels in knees, together have a patient base that includes Monica Seles, Martina Navratilova, Greg Norman, and a trail of world class skiers, including Phil Mayer, Picabo Street, and Tommy Moe. In addition, when a World Cup soccer player injures a knee, there is a good chance that he will soon be on a plane to Vail to save his professional career. Interestingly, however, Dr. Steadman uses the patellar tendon method in his ACL repair. In either method, the strength of either the hamstring or patellar tendon is compromised after surgery. Dr. Steadman feels that the patellar tendon makes a better replacement for the ACL long term, and over time the weakened patellar tendon strengthens back to its original performance level, as does the hamstring.

Another explanation from those surgeons who advocate the patellar tendon method is that the hamstring plays a crucial role in stabilizing the knee joint when the body is forced to do abrupt and severe lateral movements, which are common in sports. Compromising the hamstring, these surgeons believe, can place further stress on the knee joint. But harvesting the patellar tendon is not without risks, as it can create soreness at the front of the knee after the ACL repair, similar to patellar tendinitis. Perhaps the critical element involved is that Dr. Steadman has perfected his specific technique related to using the patellar tendon in ACL repair, just as Dr. Garrett has perfected his technique using the hamstring. Consequently, rather than basing your choice of surgeon on whether he or she uses a patellar tendon or a hamstring for the ACL repair, you would be better advised to base the decision on how many knee surgeries the surgeon has done—and other issues that are covered in Chapter 8.

Case Study: Repair of the ACL

Kevin Case of Atlanta suffered from a sore knee for more than a dozen years. In college he was an active football playing athlete

Ironically, it wasn't football that injured his knee, but rather a particularly aggressive basketball game he played while still in his twenties. While rebounding under the backboard, one of his legs got tangled in with another player's. The pop that he heard, and the subsequent agony he felt, was probably his ACL tearing. Over time, Kevin was able to get back to playing mixed doubles tennis with his wife. He was able to stay active for about ten years. Unfortunately, in 1998 while scrambling backward to hit an overhead, he felt the knee buckle under his weight. Tennis was over for a while. After hobbling around for several months, he was convinced that this injury was not going to improve without surgery. The examination revealed that Kevin's anterior cruciate ligament was badly torn. Given his athletic lifestyle, surgery would be necessary to repair it.

Repair of the Anterior Cruciate Ligament

1 *Step 1: Get ready for Day Surgery: Many knee centers have their own surgery suite. Because ACL reconstruction is a relatively quick procedure, most are done on an outpatient basis, Kevin and his wife arrived for surgery in the morning and went home that afternoon.*

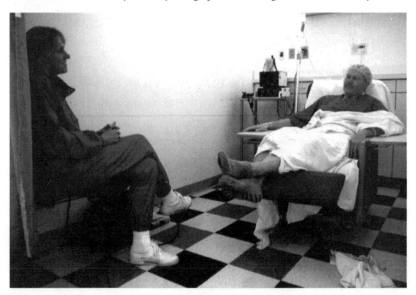

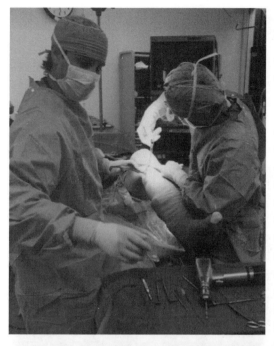

For a proficient surgeon who has done hundreds of reconstructions, the procedure rarely takes longer than an hour and involves few surprises. Kevin's leg is held by a device to keep it in position during surgery. The procedure starts with a two-inch incision at the top of the shin, just below the kneecap. This opening, and two other small ones for the arthroscope, will provide adequate access for the repair of the anterior cruciate ligament. A hole is drilled through the shin bone, and then upwards through the knee into the femur. The new ACL is threaded from the shin bone, up through the knee joint, and then into the femur.

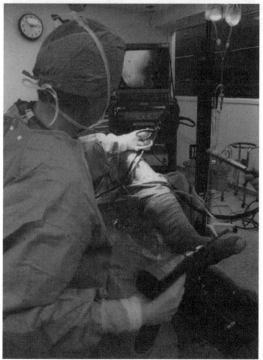

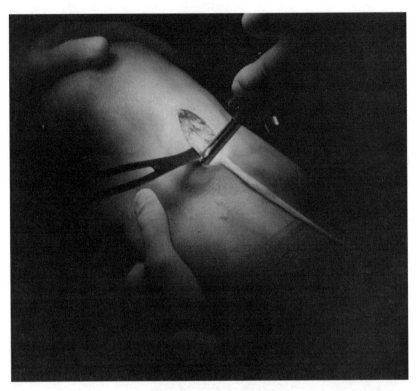

Step 3: Harvesting the new ligament. Kevin's torn anterior cruciate ligament will be replaced with tissue from his own body, in this case two tendons. The tendons are removed from the thigh by inserting a wand-like instrument through the incision site up at the shin.

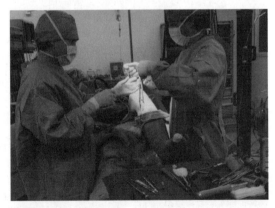

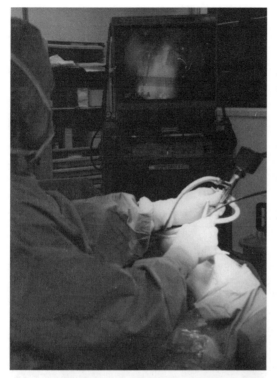

Step 4: Cleaning up the knee joint. The surgeon uses an arthroscope to remove the remnants of the torn ACL, while a surgical assistant prepares the harvested ligaments (shown below). The two eighteen-inch long hamstring tendons are doubled over to form four strong strands: the new anterior cruciate ligament.

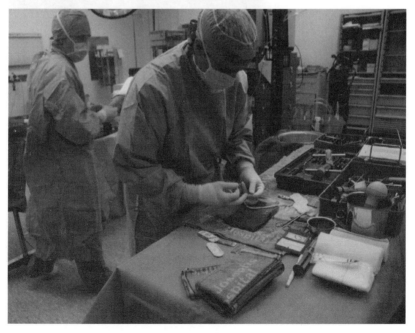

Step 5: Preparing the new ACL. The photos on these two pages show the surgeons preparing the replacement ligament harvested from the thigh. One would think that since the original ACL was only *one strand, and the new ligament is four strands (two long ligaments, doubled over)* the new ACL would be stronger. *Unfortunately, that is not the case. After implantation the grafted tendons reform, diminishing in strength to* about 60 percent of the original *ACL. Sadly, surgery cannot fully reproduce the characteristics of the original ligament.*

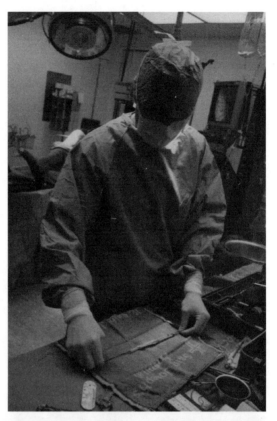

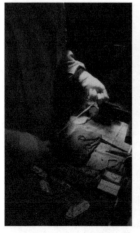

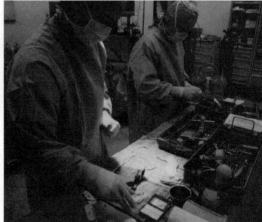

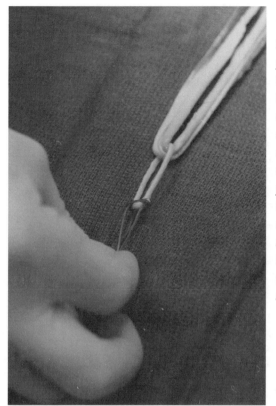

6

Left, the new ACL. The next few steps illustrate how the ligament is anchored in place. Below, the ligament is threaded through the incision in the shin area, up through the tibia, across the knee joint, and then into a hole drilled through the femur (thigh bone). Once the hook passes through the femur, it is flipped perpendicular against the bony structure. The hamstring tendons are looped through a sling which is attached to a device.

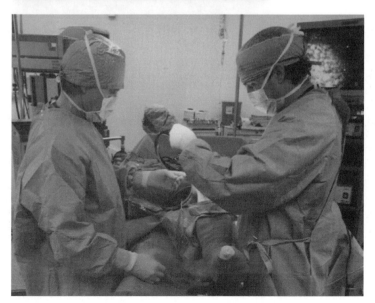

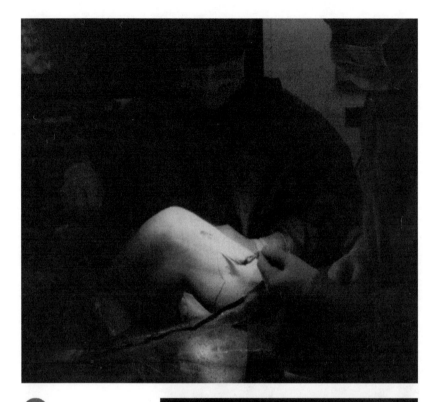

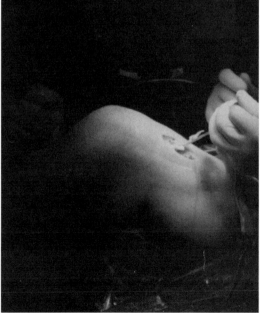

7

Top, the surgeon pulls the newly fabricated ligament up through the hole drilled in the femur (thigh bone). Bottom, the new ACL is anchored into place on the femur, then the other end, and is pulled snugly through the tibia. The bottom end of the ligament is anchored to the tibia (shin bone) with a screw.

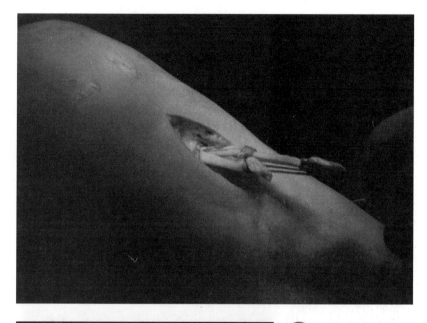

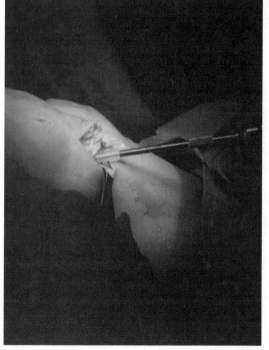

8

The final step in the surgery to replace a torn ACL: securing the new ligament in place. This is accomplished by pulling the replacement ligament down through the hole drilled through the shin bone and then screwing in a plastic dowel that locks the new ACL into the hole. Over time, the bone and the ligament, originally harvested from the hamstring, will grow together. Kevin will awaken from anesthesia within thirty minutes and leave for home within a few hours.

What Level of Activity Can Be Expected
after ACL Surgery?

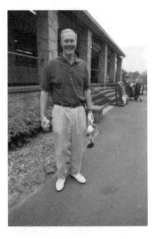

Physicians differ in their recommendations for activity after ACL reconstruction. Some warn against sports like basketball, which require lateral movement.

For example, ACL patient Kevin went back to work quickly, within a couple days. But he was instructed to take it easy with sports activities at first.

Generally, he limited himself to walking around the lumberyard, which he manages and construction sites at client locations. While his favorite sport is tennis, Kevin didn't want to jump back into heavy lateral movement too quickly. With the memory of his initial injury fresh in his mind, he didn't want a major setback.

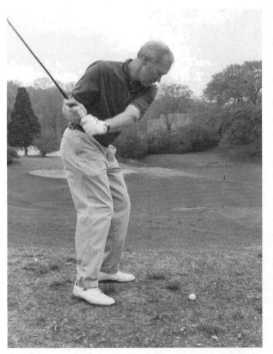

Two months after surgery, Kevin started playing golf, quickly working back to this normal scores in the nineties. By month three, he was starting to hit tennis balls on the court. Only at five months after a full rehabilitation was he allowed to return to sports without restriction. However, that thinking may be dated. If a patient is motivated to rehabilitate and uses common sense about lunging, there is no reason he or she shouldn't be able to return to sports after reconstruction.

Repairing the Permanently Damaged Knee Joint with "Total Knee Joint Replacement"

Over time, arthritis can degrade knee function to the point where medical treatment and arthroscopic surgery are no longer effective.

Those suffering from severe arthritis may have such restricted mobility that they are limited to walking distances as short as a block or two and standing for periods in excess of a quarter of an hour becomes nearly impossible. Eventually pain hampers all activities.

Work, especially that which requires prolonged standing, bending, and stooping, becomes impossible. Standing at the stove, cooking, grocery shopping, and heavy housework become difficult. As disability progresses, patients often restrict activity. Being less active, they burn fewer calories and as a consequence gain weight, placing ever-increasing loads on weak, sore knees. Eventually, these individuals come to total knee replacement.

Because the press tends to sensationalize advances in medicine, news articles create the false impression that if someone ruins their knee joint, they need simply to go to the doctor for a new bionic joint, which is better than the original. That is far from reality. Unfortunately, medicine is unable to recreate the normal knee. The knee you were born with was an engineering masterpiece. When it was working well, it allowed you to run for hours, up and downhill, and turn and twist—all without complaint.

The goal of total knee replacement surgery is to reduce

pain and to increase mobility, thereby restoring function. The overall aim is to restore a person to a comfortable and reasonably active life.

Total knee replacement surgery is utilized only in extreme cases of arthritis, in which other simpler forms of treatment have failed.

Is Knee Replacement a New Procedure?

Total knee replacement has been performed for the past thirty years and considered a successful type of joint replacement, similar to that which is performed on the hip.

Each year, about 250,000 total knee replacements surgeries are done in the U.S., according to HCIA, a Baltimore-based health information company that tracks hospital statistics.

Who Is the Typical Person Who Needs Their Knee Replaced?

Interestingly, the number of knee replacements is increasing by about 4 percent a year, perhaps because the front end of the baby boom population—those people born between 1946 and 1964—are approaching retirement age.

The average age of a total knee arthroplasty patient is sixty-eight. While many people in their fifties might benefit from a knee replacement, most doctors will try to extend the function of the original knee as far as possible.

This is because a knee implant is only good for fifteen or twenty years. A few people undergo knee replacement in their forties as a result of trauma. Less than 1 percent of knee replacements are done on patients under forty years old. Of those people undergoing knee replacement, 64 percent are covered by Medicare. About 65 percent of total knee replacements are done on women.

The surgery itself can be done in less than two hours. A total knee surgery patient will typically spend about four or five days in the hospital. According to HCIA, 57 percent of patients undergoing their first knee replacement go home afterward to begin rehabilitation. About 23 percent have to go to a skilled nursing facility for after care.

Who Should Consider Total Knee Joint Replacement?

For an orthopedic surgeon to recommend a knee replacement, the pain and extent of a person's disability must be severe. A good surgeon will be pragmatic about the limitations of the artificial new joint and will try to delay the procedure for as long as possible, since the life span of an artificial joint is limited to about fifteen or twenty years. After that point, the surgery must be repeated to replace metal parts.

Most surgeons are reluctant to implant an artificial knee much before sixty years of age. The longer the initial surgery may be delayed, the better. Thus, many surgeons encourage perseverance, use of anti-inflammatory medications, mild analgesics, and even the use of a cane or walker. Typically, it is only when function has deteriorated markedly that the surgeon and patient decide to proceed with joint replacement.

However, there are a few patients, who despite their youth, have such severe knee problems that nothing is gained by prolonging the agony. This may occur with rheumatoid arthritis or joints damaged badly from trauma.

Surgeons must weigh the health and disposition of a patient. The patient with heart and lung disease may be a poor candidate for the surgery. Diabetes increases the risk of infection. Patients who are extremely overweight place undue demands upon a knee.

A person with this condition will more quickly destroy the implanted knee than someone of appropriate weight for their height. Consequently, a physician might recommend a weight loss program so the success of the surgery is not compromised.

Some individuals will attempt extreme athletics despite the warnings of their physician. Men may be more prone to abusing the implanted knee after surgery than women.

It's also not unusual for a person with arthritis to have two bad knees. Depending upon the patient's condition, both may be replaced simultaneously.

Is the Selection of the Surgeon Important?

While many orthopedic surgeons are proficient in simple knee arthroscopy, total knee replacement is often best left to those who do a large volume of such procedures.

Total joint surgery involves many variables including the selection of the implant, methods of installation, setting proper alignment of the limb, restoring reasonable ligament balance, and guiding rehabilitation.

A good outcome requires extensive knowledge and technical expertise. Similar to an experienced carpenter who knows how to hang a door properly so that it swings in balance and perfect alignment, so the expert surgeon must make decisions during knee replacement which will determine how mobile a patient will be afterwards.

For this reason, many individuals seek out centers of excellent reputation with surgeons who specialize in joint replacement surgery and perform hundreds of such procedures each year.

When it comes to complex medical procedures, practice makes perfect. Just as the U.S. Government is using volume thresholds to steer individuals away from those doctors who lack proficiency in heart surgery, anyone considering total knee replacement surgery would be well advised to seek those surgeons who specialize in and perform a minimum of one hundred knee replacements a year.

Chapter 8 provides a list of those hospitals in the nation that report the largest numbers of knee replacements.

Hospitalization and Rehab

Patients typically spend three to five days in the hospital. They are admitted the morning of surgery and undergo an operation lasting one to two hours.

Rehabilitation typically begins the following day. Patients are encouraged to lift their legs and bend their knees within limits of pain. Exercises are tailored to the abilities of a given patient.

During the first few days, therapists may move the joint carefully through a range of motion, perhaps starting at forty degrees and working up to ninety degrees, then beyond. By the second day, patients are encouraged to place their full weight on the new knee and take steps with the aid of a walker or crutches.

While there may be some pain after surgery, it's best to get moving shortly after surgery, even with some discomfort. Typically, within one to two days, patients are able to get out of bed with minimum assistance and walk distances of fifty to one hundred feet.

If a spouse or family member is available, patients typically elect to return home immediately from the hospital. Others, lacking this help select a rehabilitation center where they stay until they have gained the strength and independence to function on their own.

A couple of weeks after surgery, most are able to walk with crutches or a walker. After several months of rehabilitation, a successful knee replacement patient should be able to climb stairs, walk without pain, and peddle a stationary bike.

Exercises directed by a physical therapist continue for a month and the rehab goal is to achieve the best possible functioning. It is important that the patient exert the best effort with the therapist to achieve this.

What Kind of Mobility Can You Expect Afterward?

About 80 percent of patients have significant pain relief after the surgery. Typically, patients with osteoarthritis function best. Those with rheumatoid arthritis may still experience some pain with weather changes.

Most surgeons discourage running, or playing any sport that would impact the knee. While the original knee is able to take the load imparted from the full body weight coming down upon it, the artificial joint is not, and would erode prematurely.

Biking is a great, nonimpact sport, as is swimming. Other suitable activities include golf, dancing, bowling, and walking. Depending upon body weight and agility, a surgeon might permit doubles tennis, or moderate recreational skiing.

Activities like running, and jumping sports such as basketball are strongly discouraged because they might cause undue wear or loosening of the bond between the joint and the underlying skeleton.

What Exactly Is an Artificial Knee Joint?

In total knee replacement the surfaces of the knee joint themselves are replaced. The ligaments are retained to stabilize the knee joint and the muscles and tendons kept to power the artificial joint itself.

To do this, the knee joint is opened in such a manner as to create minimal damage to the muscles and ligaments. The bony surfaces themselves are resected with a cutting saw and nine to ten mm of bone is removed from the end of the femur and a similar amount from the upper end of the tibia, as well as under the surface of the patella.

These surfaces are then shaped in such a manner as to receive the artificial joint, which is shaped to resemble the normal anatomy of the knee, albeit in somewhat modular form.

The femur is replaced with metal. The upper end of the tibia is replaced with plastic, as is the under surface of the knee-cap. This combination of metal and plastic results in a joint of minimal friction which is guaranteed to have the best wear possible.

Joints are often cemented into place to secure fixation to the underlying bony skeleton. In some cases, especially in the younger population group they may be left uncemented, but implanted with surfaces that encourage bony ingrowth, which is a second means of securing fixation of the artificial joint to the underlying skeleton.

The Total Knee Joint Replacement Surgery

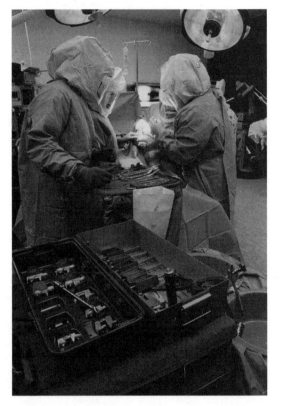

While *every operating room is sterile during surgery, compared to other surgeries, even greater care is taken for total joint surgery. Because complications of a bone infection can be severe, surgeons wear space suits with masks that protect the environment from airborne particles. During surgery, the patient is under complete anesthesia and is unable to feel any pain. The surgeon begins by making an incision to expose the knee joint fully. Shown in the foreground is some of the hardware used by the surgeon during the surgery. A surgeon may choose from several different instrumentation systems for a knee joint replacement. The selection is dictated by the surgeon's proficiency with certain systems, and which system is more suitable for a given patient.*

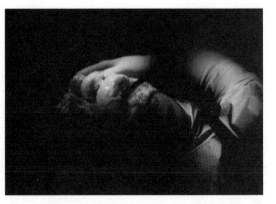

In the photo on the right, the bottom of the femur (thigh bone) is visible. After exposing the joint, the surgeon will flip the kneecap back and begin preparing the bottom of the femur and top of the tibia for the implantation of the artificial joint.

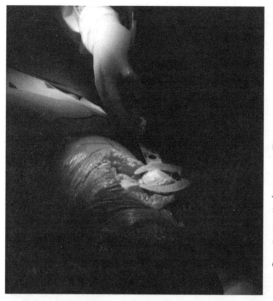

Left, the surgeon will measure the original kneecap before preparing it for a new artificial one, which will glide better over the new artificial joint.

Below, holes are drilled into the femur and the tibia, and alignment guides are used to direct the cuts made within the bone. This assures proper alignment of the overall limb.

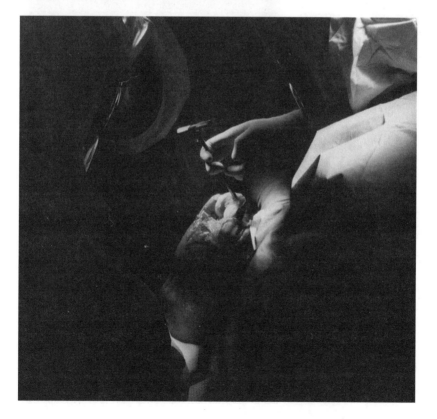

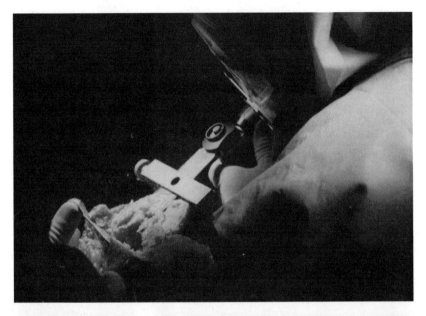

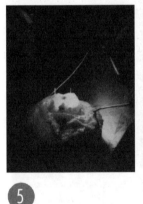

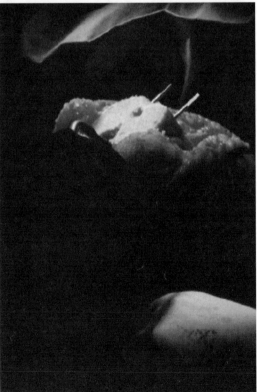

5

Top, the surgeon uses a special saw and alignment guide to precisely shape the bottom of the femur to receive the metal fitting. The metal pins shown above and on the right are guide pins providing for perfect alignment of the metal fitting. The pins are removed later in surgery after the implant is cemented in place.

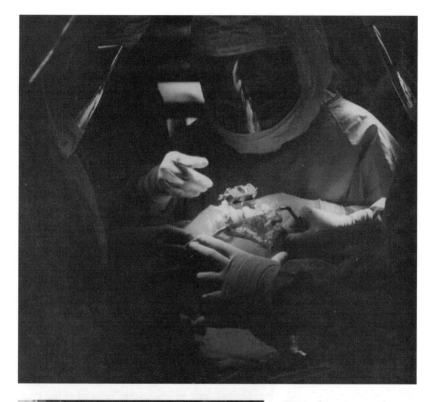

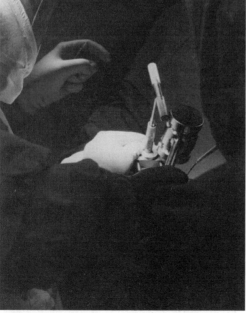

Top, Dr. Garrett sets the alignment and position of the metal fittings on both the femur and the tibia. Left, special guides are attached, and a gentle tap of the hammer secures the metal fitting snugly into its proper position.

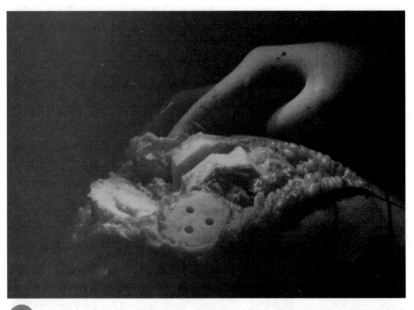

7 *The photo above shows the top of the tibia shaved flat, the bottom of the femur shaved and shaped to accept the implant fitting, and the kneecap shaved flat to accept a plastic fitting, which will form the new inner part of the kneecap. Trial parts are used to assure that the shape and alignment are proper. The final parts are coated with cement and implanted. Below, Dr. Garrett has the fittings prepared with adhesive, which will bond them to the bone.*

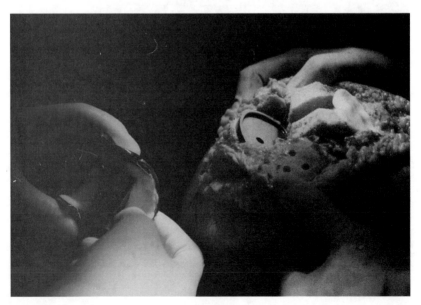

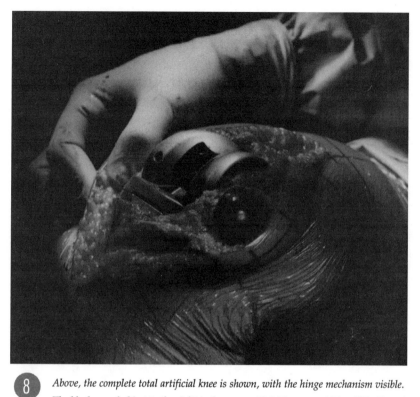

8   *Above, the complete total artificial knee is shown, with the hinge mechanism visible. The black round object to the right is the new artificial kneecap which will be flipped over into position on top of the new artifical knee joint.*

What Level of Activity Can Be Expected after Total Knee Joint Replacement Surgery?

Paul had always enjoyed an active life. He played college football for Illinois and throughout middle age Paul remained active. In his fifties, Paul played singles and doubles tennis at least three days a week. However, his aging knees became more and more painful. By the age of sixty-two, he stopped tennis and gave up his daily two mile walks with his dog. It became a painful struggle just to walk short distances. Quality of life was markedly diminished.

During the surgery, both of Paul's knees were replaced with artificial knee joints. Six months after surgery, we caught up with him as he was finishing up a couple sets of doubles tennis. On the day of his interview, he apologized that he didn't have much time to spend with me, because he was packing and leaving within the hour for the airport. He was flying to Colorado to go skiing with his grandchildren. While he planned to keep to the intermediate blue slopes, he was excited about how his new knees were performing and delighted to have a second lease on life. Is skiing too ambitious a goal after total knee replacement? And what does a surgeon think of his patient strapping two boards to his feet for the purpose of hurtling down a mountain?

Surgeons may have different opinions about how active a patient should be after knee surgery. Because of how the implant is permanently fixed to the bone, an artificial knee cannot be replaced easily. Similarly, excess demand on an artificial knee may cause its parts to wear out. As mentioned before, the implant has a life span of perhaps twenty years, and the procedure can be repeated only with difficulty. So it is not one that can be done repeatedly.

That's why some surgeons advise patients to be satisfied with activities such as walking or playing golf. Some allow doubles tennis and skiing, but most surgeons steer patients away

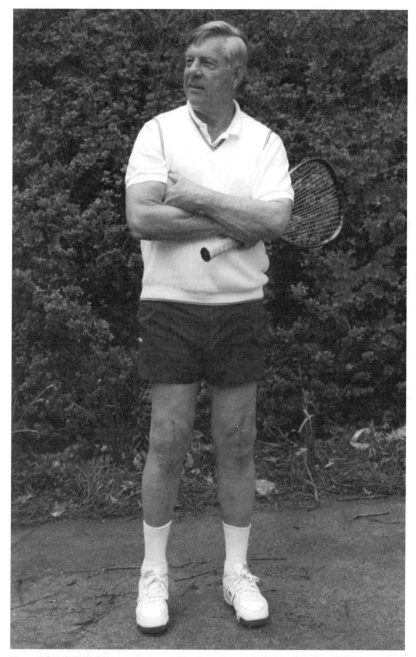

Six months after total knee replacement, Paul's knees are still puffy. The long scars are a small price to pay. For Paul, the artificial knee joints gave him back his active lifestyle, including doubles tennis. The day this photo was taken, he was leaving for Colorado to go skiing with his grandkids.

from any risky activity, such as running or basketball. No surgeon wants to see an implant damaged by an injury. But on the other hand, attention must be paid to the role of sport in the physical and emotional welfare of the patient. It's relevant to remember that life isn't a dress rehearsal. You only have one shot, and there's something to be said for enjoying it. For people like Paul, anything that a surgeon can do to restore an active life is worthwhile.

What Activities Are *Not* Recommended for Artificial Knees?

No patient with artificial knees should return to running or jogging. Doubles tennis may be okay, provided the patient is serving, or playing the net. Points in doubles often go quickly, and they are usually played out at the net with volleys rather than groundstrokes involving lots of running. The running motion is simply too devastating to the mechanics of the artificial knee joint. Plastic and metal components cannot tolerate the shock of our trunks repetitively pounding down on these joints.

Skiing may not be as dangerous as it sounds. That's because some experienced skiers can ski for three or four days without falling. Because of their skill and experience on the slopes, they may be at more risk of tripping on icy steps. In reality, for an experienced skier, skiing down an intermediate slope, provided that moguls and risky areas are avoided, may not be as damaging to the knee joint as running or jumping sports. Skiing, to the extent that the person is a proficient skier, may be permissible.

So for Paul, his total knee replacement returned him to an active life, similar to that which he had in his healthy initial years after retirement. However, Paul doesn't play singles tennis anymore, and he has had a talk with his doubles partner.

Previously Paul was the one who chased down the lobs. Now, however, that job belongs exclusively to his partner. That is part of their deal.

What Does a Total Knee Replacement Cost?

Of those people undergoing knee replacement 64 percent are covered by Medicare. Good for you, because the cost of a total knee replacement when taking into account the surgeon, the anesthesiologist, the hospital, and physical therapy afterwards, can approach $25,000.

Within the health care system, hospital-based procedures are called DRGs, which stands for Diagnosis Related Groups. This system assigns a DRG number to most things that take place within a hospital.

Here's how it would break down if you were paying out of pocket, and what Medicare pays the physician and hospital. Keep in mind, these prices are average figures.

Procedure: DRG 209 Total Knee Replacement

	Cash price	What Medicare pays
Surgeon	$5,000	$2,000
Anesthesiologist	$1,000	$600
Hospital	$14,000	$10,000
Rehabilitation	$3,000	$1,000
TOTAL	$23,000	$13,600

Knee Implant Surgery: The Second Time Around

If you have had a knee implant surgery already, and are facing revision, either because of wear or loosening of the attachment to the bony skeleton, previous concerns about choosing a proficient surgeon become even more critical.

As you might guess, when you remove the initial implant there is less bone left to work with, and in turn the surgeon has to use a bigger implant to make up for what has been removed. All of this underscores why the surgeon tries to delay the initial surgery as long as possible.

Even so, there are centers that do a large number of knee implant "revisions." Studies have shown that revisions account for one in five surgeries at large regional referral centers. In these causes, the patient have learned that it was worth travelling for the best possible result.

Advances in Knee Treatment
Coming in the Next Ten Years

In terms of research and development the 1970's was the decade in which knee replacement was formulated for people with advanced arthritis. The 1980's saw the introduction of minimally invasive surgery, with the development of the arthroscopic approach for treatment of tears of the menisci. The 1990's brought the widespread use of the arthroscopic technique for ligament reconstruction, especially of the anterior cruciate.

What Innovations Are Being Developed
for the Year 2000?

Replacement of missing parts with biologic rather than bionic material is the growing tendency. This involves repair of major holes in the joint surface and replacement of menisci. This has been driven by the need to better restore joint mechanics in the young, so the chances of developing arthritis as early as middle age are minimized.

Joint Surface Replacement

Loss of large portions of the joint surface often occurs with trauma and occasionally with developmental disorders such as osteochondritis dissecans. When it does it leaves craters in the joint surface with raw exposed bone. Patients suffer pain, stiffness, swelling, and a popping sensation within the knee. Left untreated, arthritis can occur rapidly. Several treatment options exist.

Abrasion Arthroplasty

The raw bony surface may be stimulated to grow a new joint surface, albeit one which is not as perfect as the normal hyaline cartilage of a natural joint surface. The bone at the base of the crater is either picked or burred. This procedure is called abrasion arthroplasty. The aim is to expose small subsurface blood vessels, which will grow into the area and bring with them the growth factors that will eventually produce fibrocartilage. Although not as durable as hyaline cartilage, this substitute often works well especially if a patient is young and the defect small. It can be performed arthroscopically and has been used for decades with reasonable success. However, the larger the hole the less likely it is to be successful.

Transplantation of Segments of a Joint Surface

OATS Procedure

Bony defects of small to moderate size can be filled by transplanting sections of the joint surface from elsewhere within the knee.

The procedure is labeled the "OATS" procedure (osteochondral autograft transplant surgery). Typically, the weightbearing areas of the femoral condyles are replaced by one or more dowel-shaped grafts from portions of the joint surface of the patellofemoral groove.

The aim is to replace more important sections of the knee joint with material from less important sections. Obviously there are limits in how much material can be removed, and therefore, how large a defect resurfaced. The procedure has been used over the past decade with reasonable success, especially in lesions of small to moderate size.

Transplantation of Chondrocytes

For larger lesions, a novel therapy has been developed by Dr. Lars Andersen of Sweden. Cartilage cells (chondrocytes) from the patient are harvested, allowed to multiple in the laboratory, and once an adequate population has developed, reimplanted into the defect.

This technology has been demonstrated to work reasonably well even with defects of moderate size, especially if they are well demarcated. Once again, the joint surface produced is fibrocartilage which is less durable than hyaline cartilage. However, such a patch is sufficient to cure a patient's pain. The long- term results of this procedure are uncertain.

Allografts

For larger and deeper defects, joint transplantation en bloc of living grafts harvested from tissue donors is a means of solving otherwise difficult problem of reconstruction. These defects in question typically are a result of trauma, often fracture. At times developmental disease, specifically osteochondritis dissecans, produces defects three to five centimeters in diameter.

Transplanted tissue comes from another human donor (the prefix "allo" means other). The process requires fresh transplants, and patients often have to wait months for a proper match according to age and size. The procedure initially was developed by Dr. Alan Gross in Toronto and has been used since 1972 with a high level of success.

Transplantation of the Meniscus

It is well known that patients who have undergone removal of a complete meniscus develop arthritis. The more meniscus removed, the more rapidly it occurs. Typically twenty to twenty-five years after complete medial meniscectomy, patients note significant arthritis with limitation of athletic activity. Eventually joint replacement is necessary. Thus, a teenager who undergoes complete medial meniscectomy, may develop significant arthritis by the age of forty. To offset this tendency, transplantation of menisci has been initiated.

The procedure was developed in Germany in 1984 by Dr. Klaus Milachowski and has been used since then in the United States. To date, several thousand menisci have been replaced with reasonable success. How well menisci will function decades after implantation is unknown.

Bowed Legs and Arthritis

Most people have straight legs. Some, however, most commonly men, have legs that are bowed. Although they may fancy themselves cowboys, the bowing gradually works against the proper function of their knees.

Bowing increases the force on the inner aspect of the knee, thereby increasing wear and causing arthritis. Individuals rarely note symptoms in their teens and twenties, but often by their thirties or forties are beset with pain, stiffness, and swelling. X-rays reveal arthritis within the inner area of the knee, the outer compartment of the knee being spared because the compression forces are actually lessened on that side. Most individuals are forced to lessen their level of activity, and many may face knee joint replacement within middle age.

The arthritic process can be slowed in part by lessening of activity and weight control. However, the bowing of the legs cannot be corrected with exercise or bracing. Surgery is the only solution. The tibia must be cut and the bone straightened. The procedure is called osteotomy (*osteo* = bones and *-otomy* = to cut).

The operation is one of significant magnitude, often requiring a day or two in the hospital and six to ten weeks of crutch walking. It occurs at a time of life when most people are gainfully employed. The time necessary for recovery is relatively long, but the long-term benefits of the procedure can be significant. The procedure was perfected and popularized by Dr. Mark Coventry of the Mayo Clinic and has been used with good success over the past fifty years.

Part 4

Staying Informed and
Injury-Free

Chapter 8

Finding the Best Knee Surgeon

There is tremendous change taking place in the health care industry. In the past, physicians performed the type of procedures they chose to perform.

If a general orthopedic surgeon were to receive a patient needing a total knee replacement, there was really nothing to prevent him or her from doing the procedure, even though that physician may only do a few every year. That's changing. The large group purchasers like insurance companies, Medicare, and employers are all starting to require that doctors do a certain number of complex surgeries to ensure proficiency, or not do them at all. Even hospitals, who typically cater to doctors, are sensitive to complication rates and are leaning more toward specialists and following written clinical protocols for better care. Lastly, consumers are taking more control of their choice of doctor and are selecting those centers that do a large number of the procedures required. Thanks to the Internet, consumers can research various knee specialists to determine who is best suited to do their knee surgery.

It is important to remember that hospitals don't do knee surgery—surgeons do. Theoretically, if one went to a reputable hospital one would think they would end up with a good surgeon. But that is not necessarily the case. You could end up with a staff surgeon who has not done a high volume of knee replacements. Part of the reason is that hospital administrators often run a hospital to keep it full. There are good doctors that may be on staff, as well as not so good ones. The hospital administrator typically is not one to run off those physicians who put paying patients in beds.

Sadly, unlike other industries with respected outside quality measurement entities, like the J. D. Powers quality study for the automotive industry, there is no national entity that is collecting volume data—by doctor—and then measuring quality on these volumes.

Part of the problem is that measuring health care quality is extremely complex, and there is no commonality between the various specialties in medicine. For example, quality of heart transplant surgery may be determined by the percent of patients who die from the surgery, which is called mortality rate. Quality of cancer treatment might be the percent of patients alive five years after diagnosis of cancer. But quality of orthopedic care is not typically life or death, but rather the *quality* of life after surgery. In the field of orthopedics, most quality efforts measure if the person can climb stairs, walk a mile, carry groceries, and other activities of daily living.

Also, simple quality measures can unfairly penalize the best centers. The reason for this is patient severity. In reality, sometimes the best centers may not have the best overall patient functional status scores. That's because over time, once the word gets out about a center of excellence in knee problems, that center will attract the worst possible knee problems from a statewide area.

Consider the following example. A generalist orthopedic surgeon may be getting all his patients from a nearby Zip code (which is the case with most hospitals) and these patients have relatively simple knee problems. Because these are simple knee problems, the vast majority may get better without surgery, and a higher percent will be able to climb stairs, walk a mile, etc. By contrast, the knee specialist across town has developed a strong reputation over many years as the best doctor to go to for knee problems. This knee specialist may see knee patients who come from 200 miles away because they were referred by generalist orthopedic surgeons who felt that the problem was too complex for them to handle. Instead of basic difficulties, these people have severe joint and ligament problems. As a result, even after treatment, the percent who may be able to climb stairs, walk a mile, etc., may be lower just because they're problems were more severe at the beginning of treatment. If you don't take into account the severity of the patient's problem at the beginning, the best doctor may appear to be worse than the generalist who is treating easy knee problems.

This makes the issue of health care quality management extremely complex and difficult to measure. But times are changing. There are more attempts to measure hospital and physician quality. One Internet site, at www.healthgrades.com, is publishing reports on health care quality.

While finding objective quality measures is difficult, this is not to say that the American health care consumer cannot find other ways to gauge quality and find a superior knee doctor. We recommend the following steps toward finding the best knee surgeon for your particular problem. Taken together, we believe you can develop a short list of the best high volume knee specialists in your geographic area.

Step 1: Board Certification

As a first step, a good way to qualify an orthopedic surgeon is to ask if he or she is board certified. Board certification typically requires a doctor to be out in practice a couple years (which would make the doctor "board eligible") and then the physician takes an exam by the Board representing his or her specialty association.

If the doctor is young (under thirty), he or she may not have had enough time to become board-certified. This should not necessarily disqualify the doctor from your consideration. In fact, a young doctor coming out of a knee fellowship from one of the stronger programs in the country might well be a more proficient knee surgeon than the older generalist orthopedic surgeon who is board-certified. On the other hand, if the doctor is beyond thirty years old, and still not board-certified, you may want to look elsewhere.

Also ask if the surgeon is a "Fellow" of the American College of Surgeons. The F.A.C.S. after a surgeon's name implies that he or she has passed a more rigorous exam within their specialty.

Step 2: Look for High Volume, Practice Specialization, and Fellowship Training

While the volume of surgery performed by a surgeon isn't the best indicator of quality and expertise, it's a great start. Just like anything else in which practice makes perfect, there is a good likelihood that the doctor has become proficient just by the sheer number of times he or she has performed the procedure. Also, medical research has proven that those doctors who perform more procedures have less complications and better outcomes. This is why the government and managed care companies are moving toward requiring surgeons to do a minimum number of surgeries in their specialty or stop doing them altogether.

Secondly, a steady and increasing stream of new patients implies that the procedures are successful, and former patients and existing managed care companies are steering additional patients to him or her.

When you call a prospective physician's office, ask the staff what percent of the doctor's patients are knee problems. Ideally, you want a physician where at least 50 percent of his or her patients are specifically knee patients.

Okay, if high volume of knee surgery is desirable, what is a good guideline for determining it? That is a two-faceted question because there is knee arthroscopy and general knee surgery, and then there is the implantation of artificial knees. Joint replacement surgery, for instance, is extremely specialized. Those physicians who do general knee arthroscopy should probably do at least 200 arthroscopies a year. This provides other time for them to manage nonsurgical knee patients, do joint replacement surgery, or fill in the other 50 percent of their practice with shoulders, hands, elbows, or ankle cases.

As to joint replacement surgery, at the high end, some of the most proficient and specialized surgeons will perform 500 total knee implants and 400 hip implants in a given year. With that said, the desirable minimum volume of knee implants per year should be more than one hundred, and ideally closer to 200. If a physician, for example, works on average fifty weeks a year, and does four knee implants per week, that would calculate to a 200 total.

One way to find out how many knee implants a surgeon has performed is to ask the physician. Typically, if a large part of his or her practice is directed to knee replacement, he or she should be readily able to provide a total. A second way to find out, or verify the total, is to inquire at the hospital where he or she operates. If you call Administration or the Medical Staff office, they should be willing to provide an answer to this question.

Lastly, some specialties offer fellowship training, which is an advanced training program, typically where the doctor works closely with a senior physician in a clinic that specializes in a certain problem. Fellowship training typically exposes the doctor to the most complex and difficult patients, as well as the most advanced techniques and treatments for these patients.

Step 3: Designation as a Knee Center of Excellence by a Health Plan or Employer

Disease management is a new buzzword among the top managers in health care across the United States. Managed care companies have learned the hard way that the best way to save money is *not* by forcing everybody to see primary care physicians. Some experts have estimated that 20 percent of health care consumers account for 80 percent of health care costs, because of expensive conditions like cancer, heart disease, asthma, diabetes, and back pain. Accordingly, insurance companies are putting new emphasis on finding those "centers of excellence" that specialize in high cost areas. Managed care has learned that obtaining the best quality care for patients is, in reality, less expensive than having a nonspecialist mismanage care, do unnecessary surgeries, and create problems due to botched surgery or treatment. While knee pain is not a large cost item for managed care, the cost of replacing a hip or knee joint is certainly a big ticket item, approaching $20,000 in some cases. Also, because the complications related to poor joint replacement surgery are severe in patient cost and clinical outcome, joint replacement is definitely on the radar screen of most forward-thinking health plans these days.

Consequently, one piece of information that is worthwhile to collect in your search is to call your health care insurance company, ask for the department of the medical director, and inquire if your health plan has designated a knee "center of excellence." Even if you have a knee problem that does not require knee replacement, it is likely that any knee center of excellence would also be highly proficient in routine knee problems as well. Case in point: In 1999, Blue Cross and Blue Shield of Texas recently designated five Texas hospitals as "Texas Blue Quality Centers for Hip and Knee Joint Replacement."

It is important to ask for the department of the medical director. In many plans, the medical director is usually the individual out in front of the organization trying to find the best providers. The medical director has the widest accessibility to medical groups and hospitals, outcome statistics, and other program features that make up a center of excellence. Unfortunately, because of the infrastructure of most health plans, it can take six months to filter the findings of the medical director down through the ranks to the customer service people. If your plan does not have designated a knee center of excellence, you should call other large health plans.

With this said, we offer a big caveat to this strategy. The value of this health plan referral will depend upon how progressive and advanced your health plan is at this time. About half of managed care plans are struggling to survive and many in this frame of mind will simply steer you to a physician on their plan who may have agreed to provide care at the steepest discount. In a sense, this recommendation may lead you to a physician who couldn't get patients any other way than by providing care at a cheaper rate than his or her peers.

Step 4: Check Any Available Lists and Subsets

Does your city publish a list of the largest group practices in your area? If so, look for any large orthopedic group practice. Typically, in larger cities orthopedic surgeons may join together in group practices, with each orthopedic surgeon then subspecializing in a specific area of the body. In a ten person orthopedic group practice, you may find that two specialize in spine, two specialize in knee problems, three specialize in arm, hand, and shoulder, and one does exclusively hip replacement surgery. When you call, ask who sees the most knee patients in a month. That's the doctor you want. In this scenario, you might not want to know who does the most knee surgery, because that may lead you to a doctor who leans too heavily toward surgery.

Once you determine what your knee problem is, and if you need surgery, then you may reconsider if the current doctor is the best surgeon to do your knee surgery based upon the type of surgery needed.

Another potential way to find a list of high volume centers, mixed with other factors like high reputation, use of technology, mortality rates, etc., is to go to www.usnews.com. For several years, *US News & World Report* has published a special issue called "America's Best Hospitals." The magazine ranks hospitals in a variety of specialties including orthopedics. In 1999, the top ten of fifty centers ranked in orthopedics were as follows:

1. Mayo Clinic, Rochester, MN
2. Hospital for Special Surgery, New York, NY
3. Massachusetts General Hospital, Boston, MA
4. Johns Hopkins Hospital, Baltimore, MD
5. Cleveland Clinic, Cleveland, OH
6. Duke University Medical Center, Durham, NC
7. University of Washington Medical Ctr, Seattle, WA
8. University of Iowa Hospitals & Clinics, Iowa City, IA
9. Brigham and Women's Hospital, Boston, MA
10. UCLA Medical Center, Los Angeles, CA

The problem again is that hospitals don't do surgery, doctors do. With the exception of the Mayo and Cleveland clinics, which both are doctor group practices that also own hospitals, the other hospitals listed have derived the reputation based on a group practice of physicians who admits to that hospital, along with hospital support systems like rehabilitation and ancillary diagnostic departments.

Within the rankings, about 188 different hospitals are listed, or about 3 percent of all the nation's hospitals, which provides an interesting subset to review. The method *U.S. News & World Report* uses to rank hospitals is a blend of subjective reputational information and objective hospital data.

Step 5: Call Any Policing Organizations for Information on Complaints or Malpractice Claims

Typically, state boards that police physician actions and consumer complaints have kept that information inaccessible. That's changing. To find out if there are numerous complaints against your prospective physician, you can query the board in your state that is responsible for governing state licensure of physicians.

Checking Up on Doctors

At this point, many state boards do not yet publish specific information on doctors related to reported problems or complaints. That means that to check a doctor's credentials, you will have to do some detective work. You can contact the Federation of State Medical Boards of the United States for starters. They can provide you with a listing of your state board and the doctors that are members of the American Medical Association and certified by the state board in their specialty, such as orthopedics.

Federation of State Medical Boards Inc.
Federation Place
400 Fuller Wiser Road, Suite 300
Euless, Texas 76039
(817) 868-4000

Step 6: Be Willing to Travel for the Best Doctor

If you are in a city of less than 500,000 people, you may also want to call the health plans in any nearby major metropolitan area to see if they have a designated knee center of excellence, or preferred knee specialists. Often, the best knee specialists can pick and choose the most desirable place to live, and that may not be a rural or secondary market. This brings up the question of travelling outside your own city to visit a knee specialist.

For your first visit, most board-certified orthopedic surgeons will be able to competently examine your knee and determine what may be causing your knee problem. This physician may do the necessary diagnostic tests like X-rays and an MRI scan to see inside the knee. In many cases, the surgeon may recommend a nonsurgical course of treatment, which may include therapy visits and some knee exercises. You may then be on your way back to activity, and your knee problem behind you. In other cases, the nature of your problem may be such that you need to have knee surgery or arthroscopy to repair a torn ligament, torn meniscus, or cartilage problem. This would then be the appropriate time to decide if your current orthopedic surgeon is the best person to do the surgery.

Generally speaking, if you go to a physician who spends 50 percent of his practice time focusing on knees, you will likely have someone who is proficient with knee arthroscopy and ligament surgery. If your problem is one that requires joint replacement, we recommend a second opinion from someone you find on your own versus a physician recommended by the initial surgeon. Also, if the surgeon recommends knee replacement surgery, you really have two questions: 1. Do you really need joint replacement surgery now? 2. Is this physician and local hospital the best place to have the surgery performed? Unlike arthroscopy, when you have knee replacement surgery the surgeon will be sawing off the bottom of your femur and the top of your tibia to fit the artificial knee. If there is a bone infection or the implant does not fit correctly, a redo surgery will be complicated.

Knee Arthroscopy Specialists Versus Knee Replacement Specialists

While many orthopedic surgeons are proficient in simple knee arthroscopy, total knee replacement is best left to those centers of excellence who do a large volume of these surgeries. That's because total joint surgery involves many variables, including the selection of the implant, methods of installation, setting proper alignment of the limb, restoring reasonable ligament balance, and guiding rehabilitation. On top of that, the hospital operating room has to be set up for joint replacement with air exchange systems and clean suits to prevent bone infection.

As you begin your search, you may find that those orthopedic surgeons who do a large number of knee implants may also do a large number of hip implants as well. In fact, there are many surgeons nationwide who specialize in just knee and hip implants.

At the risk of generalizing, sometimes those doctors who do a high volume of arthroscopy and surgery to repair ligament, meniscus, and joint problems, also tend to do a large volume of knee replacements. But that may not always be the case. Some knee specialists may prefer not to do joint replacement surgery, and may refer it to another orthopedic surgeon, often in the same group practice, who specializes in joint replacement. In any event, the knee specialist is often in the best position to make an informed recommendation if you need knee replacement.

Where Are the High Volume Hospitals for Total Knee Replacement?

Because hip implant surgery is often grouped with knee implant surgery, annual statistics from Medicare lump the data together. According to *Orthopedic Network News*, which summarized the Medicare data, the hospital that performed the most hip and knee implants was the Hospital for Special Surgery in New York with total of 2,744 hip and knee implants done in 1997. In second place, with 2,456 hip and knee implants was Rochester Methodist Hospital in Rochester, Minnesota, which is where the world famous Mayo Clinic operates. In ninth place was another well-known brand name in health care, the Cleveland Clinic in Cleveland, Ohio, with 1,071 total hip and knee implants. Not surprisingly, because of the large percentage of retirees, the hospitals in Fort Meyers, Florida and Fort Lauderdale, Florida were ranked sixth and eighth, respectively. It's a good idea to spend a lot of time and effort selecting the best surgeon with the highest volume of knee implant surgery. Beyond that, it is not a good idea to concern yourself with the hardware used. That's because there are more than 100 possible implant devices available, most of which are acceptable. What you desire is a return to mobility, and the surgeon's expertise with a specific type of implant is more important than the specific implant selected. In many cases, those who specialize in knee implant surgery have about five favorite knee implants. The surgeon is the best person to decide—based on all of his or her experience—which implant to use for you and your situation. Lastly, by using a certain implant model over and over again, the surgeon becomes extremely adept with it in surgery, and knows what to expect in movement afterward. So, in a sense, you are the beneficiary of all of the experience and expertise the surgeon gained from treating his or her previous patients.

Step 7: Access the Internet

The Internet is so important for the consumer, both for finding a doctor and for general knowledge about your health care problem, that we devoted the whole of Chapter 11 to the subject.

If you don't have a computer, get one. Then get on line. If you have to enter the health care system, enter it armed with knowledge about your particular problem—even before you visit the doctor. That way, you'll be sure to get your money's worth. You will be able to ask the right questions, you'll know in advance what your doctor may be looking for during the examination, and why he or she may recommend various treatments. Rather than being a passive consumer, you will become an active, inquisitive consumer who is eager to take responsibility for his or her own health—which also makes you a better patient.

Chapter 9

How to Prevent Knee Pain

Since this chapter is devoted to sports and your knees, it begs the question, "Should I even bother with playing certain sports with a bad knee, or take the risk of knee injury if my knees happen to be healthy?" We believe playing sports are a great way to stay in shape. Also, generally speaking, exercise is like a lubricant to your joints. Even people who suffer from joint degeneration caused by arthritis can benefit from movement in the joint.

When you were a kid, most of your waking hours were spent playing. As we get older, and we begin to earn a living during the week, we sometimes forget that we still need the relaxation and stress relief provided by play. Sports are a great way to do that for yourself. Sports are also a great way to keep excess weight off our frames. As we get older, the metabolism slows down, so that even while we eat the same amount and type of food our bodies need less calories, and the excess becomes fat. Too much trunk weight spells real problems for the knees. Fact: One of the best predictors of whether you will wear out your knees toward old age is if you are obese. The knees are simply not designed to haul excess weight around, especially not with the impact of that weight slamming down bone on bone. By playing sports, you keep your metabolism up so it can burn off fat. So stay lean, fit, and maintain a proper weight. Less weight on your knees means fewer knee problems down the road. It is all cause and effect.

Now, should you participate in certain sports considering that you have knee problems? In this chapter we will outline what knee injuries are common to certain sports and how to lessen your risk of developing them. Even sports like skiing, which can be one of the most traumatic sports to a knee, can be enjoyed by people with sore knees. Remember our case study patient who had just undergone surgery to implant two artificial knees journeyed back to the ski slopes of Colorado. You can too.

While we can't cover all sports, we will cover most of the favorite sports played by adults. If you are wondering about activity and knee pain, consider that your life isn't a rehearsal for something else down the road. Go have fun now, but take the following recommended steps, and be careful.

Preventing Knee Injury from Skiing

Each year, 137,000 skiers go directly from the slope to the emergency room, the majority of these trips caused by knee injury. On average, about thirty-four people die each year from skiing, according to the National Ski Areas Association. While occasionally there is a fatality, usually from hitting a tree or other stationary object while at high speed, the vast majority of ski injuries are related to knee or wrist injuries from falling.

Snowboarding Versus Skiing

Okay, you love getting away to the mountains to enjoy skiing, but you are nervous about knee injury. If you are still relatively young, in your thirties or forties, consider a snowboarding lesson.

The Rochester Institute of Technology, in New York State,

has studied knee injuries from skiing since the 1970s. They found that the most common cause of injury was from twisting and bending during falls. While skiers typically blew out their knees, snowboarders were more likely to hurt their wrists while trying to break the impact during a fall. This is not to say that you won't hurt your knees if you snowboard, just that most snowboard injuries involve the wrist rather than the knee. Snowboarding is still demanding on the knees. But on a snowboard, your feet are anchored in place, so you fall with the

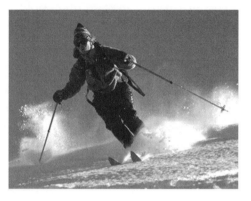

board and it doesn't come off. When you ski, you have a long six foot board attached to the bottom of each foot. When you fall, those two long boards become propellers that slam against the ground, causing a corkscrew twisting effect on your legs.

Skiing is perhaps the most brutal and demanding noncontact sport for knees. The knees are required to absorb shock from bumps and to turn the body. Inability to turn the body causes the skier to gain too much speed, which inevitably ends up in a disastrous fall. Unlike other sports such as tennis, golf, or even basketball that often result in knee injuries involving ligament strain, skiing introduces the element of bone-breaking trauma.

It is not unusual for a skier to tumble four or five times down a slope before stopping. In the process of these tumbles, the knee must resist the torque of six-foot long boards banging into the snow. Should the skier be lucky enough, the ski bindings should release with the fall and the person can tumble to a stop.

Equipment Considerations

On the plus side, there is a lot a skier can do to lessen risk of knee injury. If you are going to buy skis, don't put all your money in the boards. Instead, invest in the best bindings. If your skis are older than five years, chances are your bindings are obsolete and need to be replaced. The newer binding technology is far superior to the relatively crude bindings of five years ago. Bindings are designed to release at the first sign of a fall, provided they are adjusted correctly. The binding senses an increase in torque from the ski going in one direction and the body going a different direction. At the critical point just before something on your body snaps, the binding releases the ski, protecting your legs. If the binding doesn't release, you spin down the mountain with your skis twisting your legs like pipe cleaners.

If you are renting skis, good for you. While the skis may look beat up, most of the popular resorts use skis and bindings that are rarely more than a couple years old. The skis may look beat-up because they are used daily by renters. Typically, ski areas have very good bindings, because they want you to come back healthy and without injury.

Okay, you've bought good bindings. That's still not enough. This leads us to the second step toward injury prevention: adjustment of the bindings. The best bindings in the world are useless unless they are adjusted correctly. A capable ski shop can adjust the settings based upon your skier ability — Type one (beginner or easy going on green slopes), Type two (more aggressive skier on blue slopes), or Type three (expert skiing, mostly black slopes). Leave the exaggerations for the ski lodge afterward. Be honest about your ski ability to the binding technician. Remember, you will sign a legal document with your decision. The settings *you* choose are crucial. If you are a good skier, and the bindings are set too loose, your skis will come off during your first turn on a blue slope. If they are set too tight, they won't release the ski during a fall and your legs will twist mercilessly.

Preparing the Body for Skiing

Whether you plan to snowboard or ski, you will put your knees through some demanding work, because your entire day will be spent with the knee joint in a flexed position. You don't ski or snowboard with your knees locked.

To really prepare for a ski trip, you should get started at least three months ahead of time. There are two areas that you must develop. One is your cardiovascular conditioning. If you are going to the mountains where the air is thinner, your heart has to be in great aerobic shape or you will simply become exhausted. Even if your muscles are in shape, exhaustion will cause you to become sloppy. Ski experts note that fatigue will erode your form and balance, which in turn will set you up for a fall and a knee injury.

To help condition your knees for the slope, we recommend all the exercises provided in this chapter. Additionally, you will notice that we also have some advanced exercises specifically geared to the rigorous demands of skiing. In addition to strengthening your knees, some of these exercises also improve your aerobic conditioning.

Avoiding Trauma

We are presenting here the common sense "Responsibility Code" from the National Ski Areas Association. The reason? Many ski injuries result from people skiing out of control and hitting objects and other skiers.

Even if you are a good skier, if you have an unwise habit of stopping to talk with friends in the middle of a run, especially just over a ridge or around a turn, you are setting yourself up for a crash from another skier. Other ski falls and collisions are simply caused by getting caught up in the excitement of going fast. The faster you go, the less control you have and the less time you have to react to someone cutting in front of you.

One last bit of advice as you embark on your ski trip. Most ski injuries happen late in the afternoon, as people become fatigued, lose their balance, and fall. If you are planning a four-day trip, and if you are a blue-slope skier, promise yourself to ski green slopes on the first day to warm up. And then, when you go up to blue slopes later on, take it easy late in the day as your legs become fatigued.

Water Skiing

Water skiing can be damaging to the back and the knees because of the constant vibration caused by the ski against the water, which creates a jackhammer effect on the body. Like the snow skier, the water skier must have knees that are comfortable in a flexed position for an extended period. The wall slides shown in this chapter can be a good exercise to prepare you for a return to water skiing.

Skier's Responsibility Code

1. Always stay in control, and be able to stop and avoid other people or objects.
2. People ahead of you have the right of way. It is your responsibility to avoid them.
3. You must not stop where you obstruct a trail, or where you are not visible from above.
4. Whenever starting downhill or merging into a trail, look uphill and yield to others.
5. Observe all posted signs and warnings. Keep off closed trails and out of closed areas.
6. Prior to using a lift, you must have the knowledge and ability to load, ride, and unload safely.

One of the key differences between the snow skier and the water skier, is that when the snow skier falls, he or she is landing on ground where the water skier has a much softer impact in water. But like snow skiing, the two separate water skis on the knee can have the same twisting effect. If you have knee problems, and are adamant about

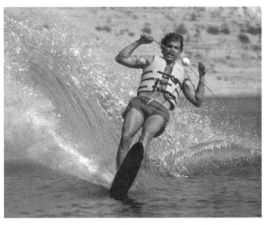

wanting to water ski, you might be better off with a single ski board instead of two separate water skis.

Basketball

Probably the most destructive sport after skiing is basketball, especially when it involves men in their thirties and forties where the ligaments and joints become less resilient to twisting and

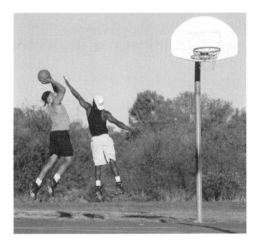

impact. The reason why basketball causes so many knee, foot, and ankle injuries is really not the running or jumping, rather it's often from coming down from midair and landing on someone else's foot, or landing off balance, which sprains an ankle or tears an anterior cruciate ligament. While basketball is not a contact sport to the same extent as football—where knee injuries occur from the abrupt forces like shoulder pads hitting the front, sides, and back of the knee during a tackle. Instead, basketball can be risky because men continue to play aggressive basketball as they get older, playing with the same intensity and competitiveness as when they were in college, though their   bodies have changed. Our ACL case study in this book, Kevin, first tore his ACL playing—yes that's right–basketball.

Football

Thankfully, tackle football is played only by young kids, high schoolers, and college players who are fairly resilient. Touch football does not generate anywhere near the problems as tackle, as it mostly involves running and cutting movements.

Still, a main element of football is to tackle someone about the legs to bring them down. This sets the stage for all types of brutal and cataclysmic, career-ending knee injuries to the MCL, LCL, PCL, and ACL. There is debate among those in football as to whether risk is increased or lessened with the type of shoes and spikes. While professional teams often play on artificial surfaces, all high schools and most colleges play on grass with spikes. While spikes increase traction while running, they also serve to lock the foot against the ground when the knee is struck from the side. But Astroturf has its own critics, including Mike Renfro, former wide receiver for the Dallas Cowboys and Houston Oilers, who suffered a severe knee injury that prevents him now from running without pain. "I hate Astroturf," he notes. "It grabbed my foot and probably caused half of the damage."

Renfro is most remembered as the player whose controversial catch at the back of an end zone in a 1980 AFC Championship game acted as the catalyst for the use of Instant Replay for officiating. During his rookie year with the Oilers, Renfro took a severe hit to his knee that tore his ACL, MCL and LCL. "Most experts doubted my return," remembers Renfro. "It took 300 days of weights, stretching, biking and swimming to return. I was a lot more enlightened about the need to take care of my knees after that experience."

Aside from being in incredible physical shape, and doing some knee strengthening exercises, there is not much someone can do to prevent the trauma that is just part of football. We don't recommend it for adults.

Soccer

Soccer is a great recreational activity, though rarely played in the United States by adults. It forces the player to be in great cardiovascular conditioning, and it requires excellent dexterity with the legs to maneuver the ball downfield. Competitive soccer does tend to cause impact injuries to the MCL, LCL, PCL,and ACL, but not as bad as football. Any of the exercises shown here in this chapter that strengthen the front of the knee and the patellar tendon, are all good for soccer.

Golf

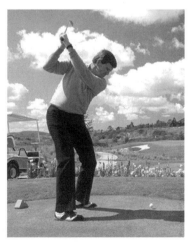

Golf is a great sport and great exercise for the knees, especially if you walk. Those with knee pain, who also want to walk for the benefit of the exercise, should probably pull a cart with their bag on it rather than carry it. Another recommended strategy: Get a small lightweight carry bag and reduce the number of clubs to ten instead of fourteen. This can make the bag easy to carry. If you don't think you can reduce the number of clubs, do this exercise: The next three times you play, on the back of your score card list all the clubs except the putter, and make a hash mark next to the club every time you hit it. You will find that the two iron, three iron, and four iron are rarely hit, or rarely are they hit well, by most golfers with handicaps of twelve or more. They could be left out of the bag, or you could reduce the bag to every other club by carrying a three, five, seven, nine, and wedge.

The second consideration related to knee problems and golf is that most people who play the game have serious form problems, which cause inconsistency and poor scores. In some cases, these swing faults include excessive lower body movement during the swing, which can place unnecessary stress on the knee. If you have knee pain that seems to get worse after you play golf, we recommend that you find a good golf pro. He or she can identify any swing motions that may be causing excessive knee rotation or side movement.

Tennis and Other Racquet Sports

While tennis is not an impact sport like skiing, football, or basketball, it generates a tremendous number of knee problems, including ACL tears, patellar tendinitis, kneecap irritation, cartilage damage, and meniscus tears. To play tennis well, the player must start, stop, turn, twist, and lunge to reach balls that are intentionally hit out of his or her reach by the opponent.

There are two general types of knee problems related to tennis. The first is overuse syndrome and it relates more to experienced tennis players who have joint problems from excessive time on the court. These knee problems show up over time with a steady ache that worsens with time on the court. The second relates to ACL tears and meniscus tears related to weekend athlete types who overdo it and come down awkwardly after a volley or overhead, tearing a ligament or a meniscus pad. To prevent the second type of knee injury while playing tennis, the weekend warrior must commit to doing some knee exercises and stretches during the week. That way, the knee will be strengthened for the weekend's activities.

Knee pain that comes on over time, often relates to degeneration of the cartilage or joint perhaps from arthritis, or from meniscus tears that worsen over time. A knee specialist is typically needed to determine what may be the source of the knee pain and if surgery can relieve the chronic pain.

Running and Jogging

As we get older, we all seem to notice that the pounds tend to creep up on us. Some of us turn to running and jogging to keep them off, and the blood pressure down. And generally speaking, running is okay for the knees, provided you don't overdo it.

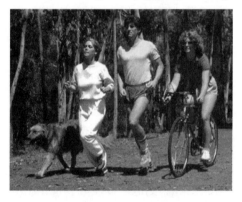

The knee problems often associated with simple jogging are typically not ligament tears, as there isn't as much lateral movement and torque as in other sports like tennis. Instead, runners can experience patellar tendinitis, hamstring pulls, kneecap pain, and meniscus tears from the up-and-down impact of bone on bone. Over time, the shock-absorbing meniscus pads just can't handle the shock, especially if the runner is overweight. This can present a quandary for the overweight person. How can you lose weight to run if you can't run to lose weight? Those people who are overweight, and are adamant about running, should consider either running on a softer track, like those found at high schools, or on a dirt trail. Running on grass can be good, except when the ground is uneven or slippery, which can cause the knee to slip or twist.

Walking

If you think walking isn't exercise, think again. Walking five miles per hour—which is a good clip—can be as good as running six miles an hour, which is a pace many joggers plod along at. In fact, running at this pace only places more shock on the knee joints. A University of Colorado study found that racewalking provided the same gains in cardiovascular fitness as running and step aerobics. The only difference was that over time, the runners tended to miss more workouts because of injuries compared to the walkers. Racewalking can also firm the butt by virtue of the stride. How fast is a five-mile per hour walk? Try walking fast. As you reach the "break-point" speed where it would seem to be easier to just run, you are now at about 4.5 miles per hour. An experienced racewalker on the other hand, can reach speeds of 5.5 miles per hour without turning into a run movement. So in a sense, you are actually working harder by staying at a walk movement rather than a run. If you walk at a 5.5-mile per hour pace, you will find yourself passing slow joggers on the path. Bottom line, part of the reason walking can be a good exercise for knees is that it is tougher on the legs than running, but does not have the impact of the body weight slamming down on the knee joint.

Biking

Another way to stay in shape is to bike, either outside or inside on a stationary bike. Because you are seated, you are removing the bone on bone impact caused by running.

The downside of biking, however, is the movement required typically involves a fuller range of motion than in other sports. A good starting exercise is the biking exercise in Chapter 6, in which you lie on your back and pedal with your feet in the air. This will help your knees work through the required range of motion without weight resistance.

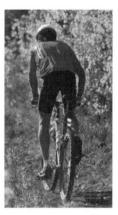

Swimming

At last we come to the least impact-oriented exercise for knees—swimming. Swimming enables the knee to move freely by kicking through the water, without any bone on bone impact, as found in running. Perhaps the only knee pain associated with swimming is suffered by those people who have kneecap pain or patellar tendinitis. The kicking motion in the water requires a bit of extension, which can cause irritation to the area of the knee.

Footgear for Sports

As with any sport that relies on running and jumping, we recommend investing in high quality shoes that are designed for the surface you are playing on. If your feet also hurt after playing, and you can't find a comfortable shoe, consult a podiatrist, a doctor who specializes in feet problems, or an orthopedic surgeon who specializes in foot and ankle. They can evaluate your foot and determine the best shoe for your needs. If you find that sometimes your ankle buckles, you might consider a higher topped shoe that can lend more support to your ankle.

The arch of the shoe can play a big role in foot problems, which may extend up to the knee over time. Do not buy a shoe based on a TV ad. Certain manufacturers gear their workout shoes for fashion versus function, because they feel people prefer shoes that don't look wide and clunky. But in reality, those tennis players who have spent years on the court will find that their feet have spread out over the years, which requires a wider toe box. These athletes may have to do extra work to find wide or EE-width tennis shoes.

If you find a shoe that is comfortable for you, we recommend that you buy three or four pair of the same shoe, same size, same width. If you are in your thirties, your feet won't be changing much. But shoes do. Manufacturers are a fickle bunch, choosing to change shoe styles frequently. When your comfortable pair of shoes wears out, you will be back to square one in the painful search for a shoe.

Knee Braces for Sports

There are dozens of knee braces on the market for knee problems. Some are designed to hold the kneecap in place, others are designed to restrict lateral movement for a weakened ACL. Before you go out and invest money in a crutch for your knees, visit a knee specialist to get his or her advice. If the doctor does recommend a brace, you will get the right one for you.

Preventing Knee Injuries in Kids

Many communities around the country are creating local ordinances that require young bikers to wear bike helmets. The new fad of roller blading, however, has created a new risk—not so much of head injury but of knee injury.

The best move a parent can make for their children who love to roller-blade is to encourage the use of both a helmet and knee pads. Many avid roller-bladers modify their skates so they can "grind" on metal poles and do acrobatics off jumps and

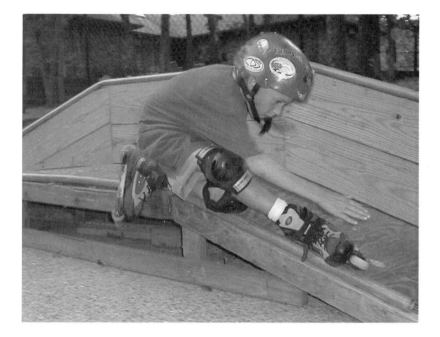

ramps. The sport has become so popular that many Colorado ski resorts have roller- blade parks during the summer for enthusiasts. These parks feature half-pipes, ramps, and jumps—all designed to get the skater airborne. When all goes well, the skater lands on the skates. There are times, however, when the youngster can come down with the bare knee breaking the weight of the body against the pavement. This can fracture the patella which could cause lasting knee problems—a keepsake of childhood.

While your kids may complain about it, a parent would be well advised to insist on knee pads for any roller-blader who is doing stunts. Knee pads aren't a cure-all, but they can protect the knee pad from fracture during many common falls.

Exercises That Make the Knee Injury-Resistant

Okay, you're ready to start moving your way back to activity. If you have severe knee pain, and you can't do all of the easy exercises in Chapter 6 without pain, then stop right now. You probably shouldn't attempt the exercises in this chapter before see-

ing a knee specialist, and letting the knee doctor circle which of the following exercises may be okay for your knee problem.

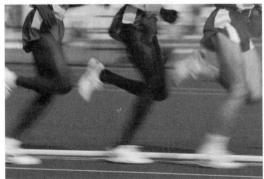

For example, those people with patellar tendinitis, or anyone who has had their ACL replaced in the last year where a piece of the patellar tendon was harvested to make the new ACL, will all have difficulty with any knee extension exercise shown in this chapter. More to the point, all of the exercises in this chapter are advanced knee exercises. Some of the advanced exercises are used by the Steadman-Hawkins Clinic in Vail to strengthen the knees of professional athletes like tennis Grand Slam champion Martina Navratilova and Olympic skiers who are recovering from knee problems to regain top form. They can be a challenge for a healthy knee, let alone a weakened one.

Trying to make a weakened knee perform advanced exercises could cause more problems. The safest route is to consult with your knee doctor and let him or her prescribe which exercises are best for you.

With those considerations and cautionary notes, here are exercises that strengthen your knees for the slopes, courts, and running paths. Remember, stop if you experience pain or discomfort.

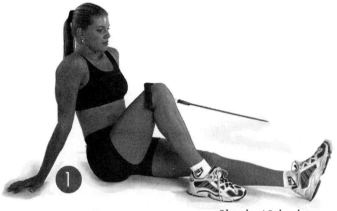

Thigh ADduction

Overview: This exercise strengthens the quadriceps muscle in the upper thigh. How to do it: Attach one end of the SportCord to a low stationary fixture, the other to the area three inches above your knee. You can also use the Sportcord belt. Slowly extend your right knee outward toward the floor. Hold for ten seconds, then return to starting position. Repeat ten times. Switch legs and repeat.

Two-Leg Minisquat

Overview: We're going to work up to a full deep knee bend. This is a one-third squat. The following exercises then go the rest of the way. You can do this exercise with the SportCord to add extra resistance. How to do it: Stand with feet together about twelve inches inches apart for good balance, and with the SportCord underneath the shoes. You can either hold the Sportcord ends in your hands, or to make it easier, hook your thumbs into your waistband. Slowly begin to lower your body, but no more than eight inches. Duplicate the position shown. Hold for ten seconds, and then return to a standing position. Repeat ten times.

One-Leg Minisquat

Overview: This exercise puts the weight of the body on single knee. You can also use the SportCord to add extra resistance. How to do it: We reccomend using the back of a chair to help your balance. Stand on your right leg with your left leg held back. Slowly, lower yourself about twelve inches to duplicate the thigh angle shown. Repeat ten times with each leg.

One-Leg Full Squat

Overview: This exercise also puts the entire weight of the body on a single knee. How to do it: Use two chairs to help your balance. Stand on your right leg with your left leg out in front. Slowly, lower yourself to duplicate the forty-five degree thigh angle shown. Do not go farther. Hold for five seconds and stand. Repeat five times with each leg, switching legs after each time. It's okay to use your arms to help you lift.

One-Leg press

Overview: This exercise will help you work up to the squat exercises, which use the body weight. In a gym, you can do leg extensions on a machine. At home, you can use a SportCord to add resistance. How to do it: Sit in a chair with the loop handle of the SportCord or belt around the instep of your shoe, not the tip. Slowly extend your right leg fully, and hold for ten seconds. Repeat ten times, then switch legs.

Ski Exercise: Balanced Stretch

Overview: Here you will work on agility and balance. How to do it: Stand and reach behind you and grasp your right foot as shown. Slowly bend forward and extend your left arm outward. Hold for ten seconds, then return to starting position and switch legs. Do ten stretches with each leg. If balancing is difficult, hold onto the back of a chair. Do not pull the foot any farther back than shown.

Ski Exercise: Half-Squats

Overview: A full deep knee bend can be tough on a recovering knee because of the full range of motion required. Work up to this with the half-squat. How to do it: Stand with feet about six inches apart for good balance. Slowly begin to lower your body, but no more than twelve inches. Duplicate the angle shown, or about a forty-five degree angle from your thigh to the floor. Hold for ten seconds, and then return to a standing position. Repeat ten times.

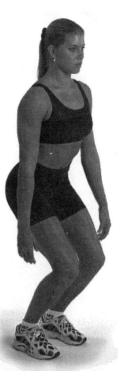

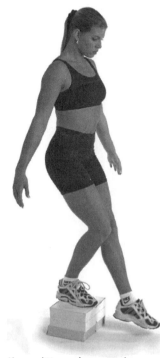

Ski Exercise: Step Downs

Overview: Stairs are brutal on sore knees because they require the knee to support the entire body weight, as the knee is bending. Skiing, especially water skiing, not only places body weight on a flexed knee, but additional weight because of the impact of the snow or water on a flexed knee. This exercise can help prepare the knee for that by balancing the body weight on a flexed knee. How to do it: You can use a stair or stack of books. Start with both feet on the platform, then extend your left leg out and slowly lower your body on the right knee. Hold for five seconds, then return to starting position. Repeat with the other leg.

Knee/Hamstring Flexion

Overview: This is an important exercise for the knee. At home a SportCord can simulate a weight machine in adding resistance to this hamstring exercise. How to do it: Attach one end of the SportCord to a doorknob, the   other to your ankle. Slowly flex your ankle back toward the chair.

Try to drag the toe against the ground. Hold for ten seconds, then repeat ten times. Switch legs and repeat.

Ski Exercise: Windmill Hops

Overview: Skiing requires great aerobic conditioning, agility, and balance. This exercise requires all the above as it rotates the upper body and works the knees with moderate impact. How to do it: Place a towel on the floor. Start on your right foot with your left hand on the floor, as shown in picture one. Next, jump upward from this position, across the towel landing on your left foot and right hand. Get momentum going and hop from side to side for one minute, then rest. Repeat for ten one minute intervals.

Ski Exercise: Deep Knee Bends

Overview: Okay, the knee exercise you've been dreading. Depending upon how aggressive you want to be on the slope, deep knee bends, with no impact, can stretch a healthy knee and condition it for the jackhammer effect the knees may get on crusty snow, or the spring action generated by fresh powder. How to do it: Start with the feet shoulder width apart and hands outstretched for balance. Slowly lower the body (don't bounce down and up) until the thighs are horizontal. Hold in the squat position for five seconds, and then stand. Repeat ten times. Not fun? Rest assured we don't know anybody who likes deep knee bends. But they do prepare the knee for the workout they will get on the mountain.

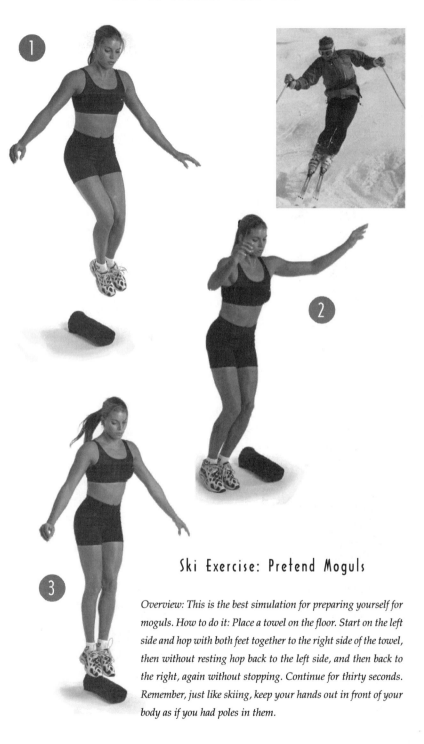

Ski Exercise: Pretend Moguls

Overview: This is the best simulation for preparing yourself for moguls. How to do it: Place a towel on the floor. Start on the left side and hop with both feet together to the right side of the towel, then without resting hop back to the left side, and then back to the right, again without stopping. Continue for thirty seconds. Remember, just like skiing, keep your hands out in front of your body as if you had poles in them.

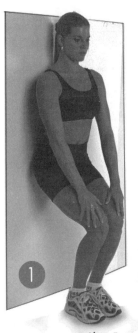
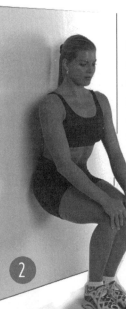

Wall Slide

Overview: For years, the wall slide has been a common exercise for competitive skiers. It places great demands on the quadriceps muscles and tendons around the knee. How to do it: Start with your back flat against the wall and your feet about fifteen inches away from the wall. Slowly slide down until your thighs are horizontal. Hold for ten to thirty seconds depending upon what you can tolerate, and slide back up. Repeat five times.

Ski Exercise: Leg Swings

Overview: This exercise requires one leg to hold the body in balance. If this appears too difficult, it can also be done with one hand holding the back of a chair. How to do it: Stand on your right leg. Extend your left leg out in front of you until it can almost touch the floor, eighteen inches out in front. Next, slowly begin to swing the left leg to the side so the leg may touch the floor, eighteen inches to the side, then back behind you, then back to start. Your left leg has made a large semicircle path from front to back. Repeat ten times, and then switch legs.

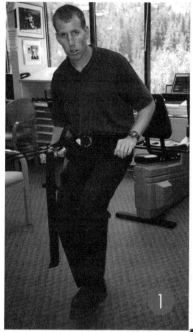

Performance Exercises for Ski and Tennis Athletes

Okay, you've made it to here. Shawn McEnroe, rehab guru for the famous Steadman-Hawkins Clinic in Vail, Colorado—which helps celebrity tennis athletes, Olympic skiers, and World Cup soccer players from around the world—shows a couple demanding exercises that get top athletes back to top form after a knee injury. These may look easy, but after five minutes your knees will feel like you've just survived a black slope. After ten minutes, you'll understand why you're not an Olympic skier.

Side-to-Side Pullbacks

Overview: This is an intense strength builder for competitive skiers. It places great demands on the front of the leg, quadriceps muscles, and tendons around the knee. It's perfect for tennis and skiing. How to do it: Anchor your Sportcord around a stationary pole, and place the belt around your waist. Sit back until the tension is holding you up and pulling you forward. Keep your knees flexed and unlocked. Now, lift off your left foot shifting all your weight to your right, hold for two seconds, then lift off with the right, placing all the weight on the left. Continue for ten minutes, if you can, never locking your knees.

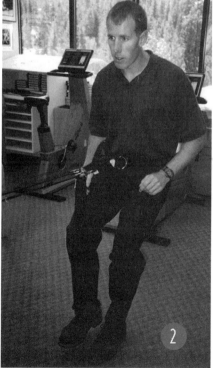

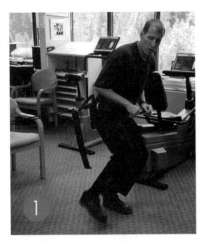

Mogul Run

Overview: Want to get a feel of skiing without the plane trip to the mountains? This exercise is guaranteed to do it for your knees. In addition to Olympic skiers using this exercise, tennis great Martina Navratilova found it helpful. She realized that she needed an extra step to cover one sideline compared to her lateral movement toward the other direction. This exercise strengthened her push off and lateral movement. How to do it: Anchor your Sportcord around a stationary pole, and place the belt around your waist. Lean outward until the tension is holding you up. Keep your knees flexed and unlocked. Now, lift off your inner right foot shifting all your weight to your left, hold for two seconds, then transfer your weight to the right foot, then back to the left. Continue for ten minutes, if you can, never locking your knees.

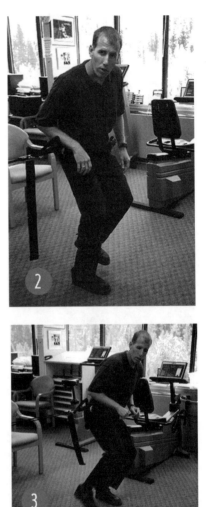

Chapter 10

How to Use the Internet
to the Benefit of Your Knees

If you have sore knees, you may find some relief at your fingertips. The Internet promises to revolutionize the health care industry. That's because the Internet is like a huge encyclopedia or medical journal that is being updated daily, with information from experts from across the world rather than just doctors from across town.

Health care is based on information. For you to receive the best clinical outcome, you must have the most current information either provided to you by the best knee expert, or you yourself must become educated about knees and what may be the best treatment.

When pain motivates you to go to the doctor, you are looking typically for two things: 1. You first want relief from your pain, which may come in the form of medication, therapy, or some other treatment. 2. You want more information about what may be causing your knee pain now, and whether it's possible to prevent it from returning in the future.

The information may come from the doctor's exam of your knee, which may also involve X-rays or an MRI scan. Other information may come in the form of dialogue between the doctor and you.

You will need a knee expert to determine the cause of your specific problem. But once you have that diagnosis, you should educate yourself as to what the best options are for you. This chapter gives you a head start in learning to use the Internet to your best advantage. So let's get started.

Search Engines

While the good news is that the Internet is a deep treasure trove of information, the bad news is that you are only able to skim the surface of the information that is on top.

The reason for this is that the most popular search engines cannot keep pace with all the new information coming onto the Internet every day. In a sense, it is like a librarian who receives a truckload of new books every day. While the information is there, no one has had time to organize it effectively.

There are ways to increase your odds of finding the information you are looking for, though. Different search engines perform better than others. *USA Today* reported in July 1999 that the popular search engines like Yahoo, Excite, and Lycos only index about 5 percent of the total content of the Internet. One of the best-ranked search engines was Alta Vista, which indexed only 15 percent of the content of the Internet.

Consequently, if you are doing a search for information on the Internet, we recommend that you bookmark Alta Vista. Here are the addresses of Alta Vista and other popular search engines:

www.altavista.com   *www.hotbot.com*
www.yahoo.com   *www.infoseek.com*
www.excite.com

How to Enter Your Search Query

Okay, you have Alta Vista, or another one of your favorite search engines, ready to do your search. How you structure your query will determine if you are continually frustrated with your results, or if the first ten responses turn up exactly what you are looking for. The key lies in understanding how the computer interprets what you type into the query box.

Keep in mind that the computer is extremely literal with the instructions you give it. The computer is not human, and cannot deduce what you are looking for.

For example, let's look on the Internet for what could be causing your knee pain. If you enter:

causes of knee pain

You will get back all those pages on the Internet that contain the following words in their sites: *causes, of, knee, pain.* You may find a worthwhile site, but it may be buried among 50 sites down on the list. Instead a better way search is to use quotation marks around the phrase you are looking for, such as:

"causes of knee pain"

Now you will get ONLY those sites where this specific phrase appears somewhere in the site. The problem with this approach is that you may eliminate a lot of good sites that have great knee information but they don't happen to use this exact phrase. Better to use the following query to look for those sites that have the specific key words, which relate to you.

+"knee pain" +causes +arthritis

Note that the use of a plus sign in front of the word is telling the computer this word is a "must have." Said another way, the above search requires the computer to only retrieve those sites that have "knee pain," "causes," and "arthritis" in their content.

Now that you know how to ask the computer to go seek out information on the Internet, try your hand with some searches and see what you find. If you don't seem to find what you're looking for, then try some of the following resource sites that we've outlined for you.

General Resource Sites on the Internet

To find a directory of orthopedic surgeons, visit the American Academy of Orthopedic Surgeons at *http://www.aaos.org/*. This site contains a listing of all board-certified members that specialize in orthopedic surgery in your area.

The Steadman-Hawkins Clinic Web site (*http://www.steadman-hawkins.com*) contains information about knee injuries and exercises, and it also contains a link to finding a good orthopedic doctor.

You can find an orthopedic doctor or surgeon by name, area, or practice through Orthoconnection at *http://www.orthoconnection.com.* Keep in mind that you then want to inquire about their level of expertise, which is discussed in our chapter on finding a doctor. Orthoconnection also contains helpful information about techniques, procedures, and general health.

Using the Internet to Find a Knee Doctor

Many people do not have the time to write various boards to locate a good doctor for their knee pain. The Internet can put information right at your fingertips very quickly.

One site you may visit is the Cleveland Clinic site. *U.S. World News & Report* ranked them fifth in terms of success rates in orthopedics. Their Web site (*www.ccf.org*) has a section on how to determine the status of doctors and hospitals.

The Cleveland Clinic Foundation notes that board certification is a good indicator of both experience and competency. In order to be board-certified, the doctor must have passed a test in their specialty area. When doctors are board-certified in their specialties, they usually have four to five years of training in that area. To retain the certification, doctors must continue their medical education throughout their careers. So generally speaking, board certification is an additional hurdle that separates experienced physicians from others who may be less qualified.

The American Medical Association (*www.ama-assn.org*) also has a link to a doctor finder that helps you locate a doctor in your area and in a specialty like orthopedics. This AMA site also provides you with detailed information on ethics and accreditation. Consumer health information is also included. The AMA site also contains FREIDA, an online service which provides information and statistics on hospitals and specialties. For example, if you were looking for statistics related to orthopedic practices and clinics, you could utilize this to find statistics on various elements of the industry.

Healthfinder is a government sponsored Web site with links that help you find a certified physician in your area. Healthfinder is located at *www.healthfinder.gov*. It also contains a link to Quality Check, a site that is sponsored by the Joint Commission on Accreditation of Health Care Organizations. It provides more detail on the quality of health care facilities and service providers, so that you can determine if your hospital or doctor meets the correct guidelines and standards. You can go directly to this site at *www.jcaho.org/qualitycheck*.

To check a doctor's board certification, you can go to *www.certifieddoctor.org*. This site is sponsored by the American Board of Medical Specialties. It contains all the physicians that are certified, and they are shown both by name and area. Those doctors that subscribe to the service have additional listings with their name that include telephone number, hospital affiliations, address, and health plan affiliation.

Other sites that will verify a doctor's credentials are *www.doctordirectory.com* and *www.mymedic.com*. These sites list doctors in your area and their credentials.

More in the area of orthopedics and knee pain, *www.orthoconnection.com* will help you search for a doctor. It also provides health tips and information on techniques and procedures related to the knee. You can ask questions and get answers from doctors who participate in this online service.

Orthopedic Avenue (*www.orthoave.com*) is another site that lists orthopedic doctors by state and gives their phone number, hours, e-mail and physical addresses.

For a complete listing of all Internet sites that relate to orthopedics, visit *www.orthoguide.com*. Orthoguide is a site that saves time by providing you with a comprehensive listing of orthopedic-related sites, which keeps you from having to search the Internet on your own.

After checking credentials, you still may be wary about a doctor's practice. The site *www.citizen.org* contains information to consider when contemplating the credentials of the doctor you are seeing.

If you are also hesitant to try alternative or complementary treatment, you may want to visit *www.quackwatch.com*. This site contains information on the latest fraudulent practices that have been discovered within the medical field.

If you are really inquisitive about a doctor's credentials and whether or not he or she has been the subject of patient complaints or state board actions, you can visit *www.americafind.net*. For $59, you can request a total background check on any doctor, and you will be provided with an extensive report regarding their education, licensing, and any actions or complaints filed against them.

For a less expensive fee, you can obtain a report from the health research group at *www.publiccitizen.org*. A regional report of doctors can be obtained for $20. The report lists the state, doctor, and the list of offenses. You can obtain general statistics and demographics on the 16,638 doctors who have had disciplinary action filed against them. For $15, a full report can be obtained on a specific doctor, and $5 is charged for each doctor report after that. The report lists the doctor's education, training, certification, and sanctions and disciplinary action taken against the doctor.

You can check to see whether a particular doctor is a member of a society or association like the Academy of Orthopedic Surgeons (AOS) by checking the site *www.a-o-s.org*. The same can be done on the American Association of Hip and Knee Surgeons (AAHKS) Web site, at *www.aahks.org*.

Our Favorite Orthopedic Sites

Here's our list of favorite sites from which you can learn more about orthopedics, knee pain, and get free tips on self-care and when to see a doctor. Some medical sites will put you on an e-mail list and send you the equivalent of a digital newsletter with current articles on various   subjects.

Orthoguide
www.orthoguide.com
This site is a search engine specifically for researching the field of orthopedics for educational institutions, organizations, research, disorders, etc.

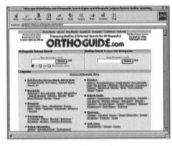

Orthogate
www.owl.orthogate.org
A comprehensive site with a listing
of physicians, clinics, and topics
about orthopedics.

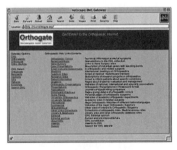

Orthosearch
www.orthosearch.com
Contains orthopedic organizations,
clinics, practices, and resources.

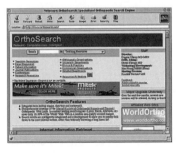

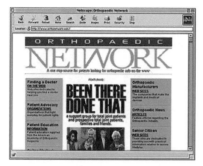

Orthopedic Network
www.orthonetwork.com
Contains recent news, guidance on how to find a good doctor, patient education and information, and orthopedic organizations.

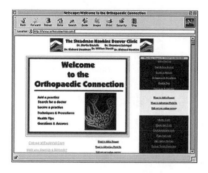

Orthoconnection
www.orthoconnection.com
This site helps you locate a practice or search for a doctor. It also provides health tips, techniques related to the knee, and Q & A with certified doctors.

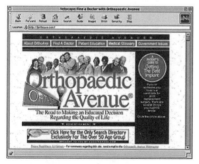

Orthopedic Avenue
www.orthoave.com
Contains information on government issues, a medical glossary, patient education, and help in finding a doctor.

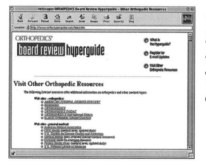

Orthopedics board review hyperguide
www.orthohyperguides.com
This site contains links to many other orthopedic Web sites.

Wheeless' Textbook
of Orthopedics
www.medmedia.com
This site is one of the first online
textbooks about orthopedics. It
also contains a listing of books,
journals, medical news, and links
to other orthopedic sites.

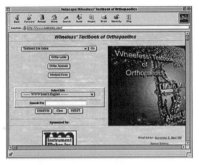

Orthopedic Internet Directory
www.slackinc.com/bone/
orthonet.htm
A guide to research and information on orthopedics.

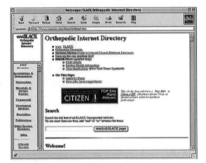

Medline Plus
www.nlm.nih.gov/medlineplus
This site has a section specifically
for knee injuries and disorders.
It has information on knee problems and treatments, and it provides directories to orthopedic
associations and organizations.

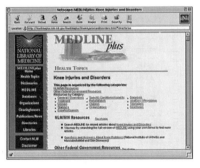

Our Favorite General Health Sites

www.americasdoctor.com
This site is a virtual doctor's house call. It provides patients who subscribe to the site with real interaction with physicians. It was originally only available to America Online Subscribers.

America's Health Network www.ahn.com
This site is related to the cable television health network with the same name. It videocasts live medical procedures on the Internet. It has been ranked as one of the Internet's top 200 most visited sites. This site has gained the most attention for filming a live birth for visitors to view.

Ask Dr. Weil www.drweil.com
This is a hot site for alternative medicine followers. Dr. Weil is a New Age physician with his own television series. Visitors to this site can ask questions and obtain information about various alternative medicine practices.

Better Health www.betterhealth.com
This site is geared toward women and focuses on fitness and general health.

Dr. Koop's Community www.drkoop.com
Dr. Everett C. Koop, the former surgeon general and well-known physician, is chairman of Empower Corp. in Austin, TX. This site offers health information, and it offers e-commerce opportunities.

DrugStore.Com www.drugstore.com
DrugStore.Com aims to be what Amazon.com has become for book shoppers. It is an e-commerce site dedicated to bringing patients drugs over the Internet, much like Amazon.com provides books.

HealthFinder www.healthfinder.gov
This government site was created by the Department of Health
and Human Services. It offers advice on just about any area and
aspect of health. It had over 1.7 million visitors in its first full
year.

Health A-to-Z www.healthatoz.com
This site is relatively new. It is a search engine specifically geared
to health-related information.

Health World www.healthy.net
This site is mainly focused on natural and alternative medicine
and self-care. It provides information to visitors on classes, journals, books, and specific information related to certain conditions. It also has shopping areas and many e-commerce
activities.

InteliHealth, Inc. www.intelihealth.com
Johns Hopkins Health Care System and Aetna U.S Healthcare
provided the content for this site. It provides health-related information, and it is a big-revenue seeker, with ad and
e-commerce activities.

Kaiser Permanente www.kponline.org
The only visitors that can access this site are members of Kaiser
Permanente's health plan. It has personal health information,
appointment scheduling, and other administrative services.

Mayo Health Oasis www.mayohealth.org
This site is part of the Mayo Foundation for Medical Education
and Research in Rochester, Minnesota. It is one of the few sites
maintained by a traditional healthcare provider. Mayo Health
has about 800,000 visitors a month.

Mediconsult.Com, Ltd   www.mediconsult.com
This site claims to have over 15,000 visitors a day. It is a virtual medicine center that offers clinical information, rather than just general information on health. This site also offers consulting and site development in addition to revenue seekers who want to profit from the site by selling advertising space or marketing consumer products for purchase (e-commerce).

My Life Path   www.mylifepath.com
This site was developed in association with Blue Shield of California to build brand awareness.

OnHealth Network Co.   www.onhealth.com
This site was designed to help consumers explore the health care system. It also provides general information on health and wellness.

PlanetRx   www.planetrx.com
This site contains health information and an online pharmacy.

Sapient Health Network   www.shn.com
Unlike other sites, which only provide general health information, Sapient Health Network has developed over fifteen virtual communities that focus on specific conditions like asthma, diabetes, depression, and breast cancer. This site also markets patient research and clinical trials to pharmaceutical companies.

Thrive Online   www.thriveonline.com
Thrive Online is the most popular consumer health site. It attracts 1.6 million visitors per month.

Your Health   www.yourhealth.com
Your Health is a public version of Access Health's online Personal Health Advisor site.

MedWeb   www.cc.emory.edu/whscl/medweb.html
This site contains one of the most comprehensive listing of medical sites.

The University of Iowa Hardin Meta Directory
www.arcade.uiowa.edu/hardin-www/md.html
Contains a listing of medical related sites that focus on consumer health, medical organizations, etc.

HealthWeb   www.healthweb.org
This site was created as a resource for people who are struggling with illness. It was developed by medical school librarians.

Medical Matrix www.medmatrix.org
Medical experts rate medical Internet sites.

MedScape www.medscape.com
A commercial site that contains very comprehensive information on general health.

PubMed   www.ncbi.nlm.gov/pubmed/
This is a U.S. National Library of Medicine site that contains a medical database of information and research.

CenterWatch www.centerwatch.com
This site provides information on how you can participate in clinical trials.

Web Sites for Researching Alternative Medicine

These sites provide the latest research and information on alternative medicine.

Office of Alternative Medicine *http://scrdp.stanford.edu.camps.html*
Health World Online *http://www.hir.com*
Holistic Healing Web Page *http://holisticmed.com*

Web Sites for Nutrition and Weight Management

www.ama-assn.org/consumer.htm
This site from the American Medical Association provides information on your diet, calculates your body mass index (BMI), and gives advice on health issues.

www.cyberdiet.com
Put in your weight, height, age, and other characteristics and get a menu, eating plan, recipes, etc.

www.dietitian.com/ibw/ibw.html
Find your ideal hip to waist ratio and a guide to caloric intake.

www.healthyeating.org
They'll calculate your BMI and assess your activity level.

www.olen.com/food
The site gives statistics on the nutritional value of fast foods.

Reviewing a Doctor's Web Site

Many doctors and group practices have their own Web sites. While many of these sites act as an online promotion for the doctor and the practice, they can provide a lot of the information you are looking for about the physician, practice volume, and area of specialization. In addition, you can get a sense of the doctor's practice philosophy, including whether he or she emphasizes surgery or a nonsurgical treatment regimen.

A Final Cautionary Note about Quackery on the Internet

Okay, the Internet is a fantastic treasure trove of information. What could be wrong with that? The problem involves promoting miracle cures for health problems. Many of these ads claim to have scientific studies backing them up to entice people to spend their hard-earned money on bogus cures.

The Arthritis Foundation is concerned about fraudulent claims of miracle cures for arthritis, which include such things as antler velvet and radioactive mineral baths.

The Federal Trade Commission also warns Internet users that many Internet advertisements are misleading to people with serious health problems. If you have a complaint about an advertised medical product, you can report it to the FTC at 877-FTC-HELP. If you are concerned about a deceptive ad, visit the FTC at www.ftc.gov or the Arthritis Foundation at www.arthritis.org.

By reading this book, you have made the first step toward recovering from knee pain. You now know what may be causing your knee pain, and whether you need to see a doctor. You also now know the things you can do on your own to diagnose your knee pain, treat it, and prevent recurrence.

The exercises can help you strengthen the knee joint and help you regain lost mobility. If you have a weight problem that is standing in your way, you now may finally have the tips and motivation you need to unburden your knees from excessive body weight. We also hope that because of this book you will make more enlightened decisions and smarter choices about which doctors to see and what advice to believe. The knowledge you've gained in this book acts as the real key to unlocking quality from the bewildering health care system. If you want high quality, demand it. Don't settle for a physician who doesn't answer the questions you ask of him or her. Go the extra distance to find the Center of Excellence with the best knee specialist available. Excellence isn't more expensive, it's the best value.

We hope the information provided within this self-help guide will help *you* back to activity and a fulfilling life. Go outside. Have fun. Remember: This isn't a rehearsal for something else.

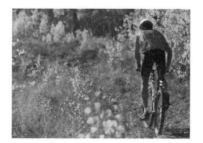

References

Bucco, Gloria. 1998. Enhancing the Benefits. *Herbs for Health Magazine.* Nov.-Dec.

Bucco, Gloria. 1998. Joint Relief. *Herbs for Health Magazine.* Nov.-Dec.

Deal, CL and R.W. Moskowitz. 1999. Nutraceuticals as therapeutic agents in osteoarthritis. *Rheumatoid Disorders Clinic North America.* 25: 2.

DeVita,P., T. Lassiter, Jr., T. Hortobagyi and M. Torry. 1998. Functional knee brace effects during walking in patients with anterior cruciate ligament reconstruction. *American Journal of Sports Medicine.* Nov.-Dec.,

Hewett, T.E, Fr. Noyes, S.D Barber-Westin, T.P. Heckman. 1998. Decrease in knee joint pain and increase in function in patients with medical compartment arthrosis: a prospective analysis of valgus bracing. *Orthopedics.* February, 21.

Jonas, Wayne B, M.D. and Jennifer Jacobs, M.D., M.P.H. 1996. *Healing With Homeopathy.* New York: Warner Books, Inc.

Keville, Kathi and Peter Kern. 1996. *Herbs for Health and Healing.* New York: Berkley Publishing.

"*MSM.*" *Total Health.* 20 (1).

Risberg, M.A, I. Holm, H. Steen, J. Eriksson and A. Ekeland. 1999. The effect of knee bracing after anterior cruciate ligament reconstruction. *American Journal of Sports Medicine.* Jan.-Feb. 27(1).

Sullivan, Dana. Sports medicine's new alternatives. *Sports Illustrated.*

Theodosakis, Jason, M.D., M.S., M.P.H and Brenda Adderly, M.H.A. and Barry Fox, Ph.D. 1998. *Maximizing the Arthritis Cure.* St. Martin's Press: New York.

Index

A

AAOS
5, 13, 50

Abrasion Arthroplasty
185

ACL
14-15, 30-31, 39, 42-43, 72, 78, 80, 86-87, 94-95, 99, 101 133, 156-166, 210-212, 218

acupressure
121

acupuncture
122-123

allografts
187

alternative medicine
19, 116-118, 121-130, 243

American Academy of Orthopedic Surgeons (AAOS)
5, 13, 50. *See also* AAOS

American Journal of Sports Medicine
15

Anterior cruciate ligament (ACL). *See* ACL

anti-inflammatories
82-82, 95-96

Arnot, Robert, Dr.
14

arthritis 5-7, 14, 38, 46-48, 88-89, 95-96, 103-106, 108-110, 119-120, 128, 172, 188, 213,

arthroplasty
185

articular cartilage
24, 41, 50,

B

basketball
40, 42, 209-210

bee venom therapy
123

biking
154, 172, 214

BMI. *See* Body Mass Index

Body Mass Index (BMI)
105-243

braces
18, 98-103, 216

bursitis
57

C

calcium
107, 111, 113

cartilage
6, 41-47, 126

chondromalacia
34, 37, 41

creatine 111-112

D

diet
9, 84, 100, 108, 116, 243

dietary supplements
97-99, 107, 120

dieting
100-108, 243

dislocation
51

doctor *See also* surgeon
seeking quality care
14-16
rating pain
37
diagnosing knee pain
62-64, 66, 68,
visiting the knee doctor
66-80,
asking about foot orthotics
99
alternative medicine
116-118
surgery
155-170
finding a doctor
170, 191-202
using the Internet to find a
doctor
232, 243

E

enzymes
97, 107-109

F

fibula
24, 48

flexion exercise
136, 148-149

football
15, 33, 40-41, 44, 88, 113, 180,
209, 211

fracture
3, 5, 34-35, 45-48, 52, 58-59,
63-64, 76, 80-82, 86, 107, 122,
178, 206

G

glucosamine and chondroitin
sulfate 108

gelatin
112

golf
10, 166, 211

H

herbs
119-121

homeopathy
123-124

hydrotherapy
125

I

inflammation
35, 41, 44, 53, 66, 76-79, 89-90,
97, 100-101, 106, 109-110,
114-116, 119

Internet
13, 18, 96, 116, 120, 125, 180, 191,
219, 220-222, 224, 228-229,
232-234

J

joint
3-5, 11, 13-17, 21-22, 24, 27,
31, 35, 42-45, 48, 49, 51, 53,
61-66, 68, 71-73, 76-79, 81,
88-93, 97-105, 107, 111, 113,
115-116, 118-119, 122-124, 126,
128-129, 131, 133, 144-147,
150, 152, 154, 158-166, 170-173,
175-179, 182-185, 189-190, 192,
196, 198, 201, 203, 234, 237

K

knee exercise
86, 122-
125, 144, 188, 207, 213

knee injuries
14-15, 19, 21, 77, 125, 145,
193-194, 198-199, 205, 222, 228

knee joint replacement
158, 160, 165, 171, 179, 185, 189

kneecap
14-15, 22-23, 25, 28-
29, 37, 38, 43, 46-47, 49, 50-
51, 53-54, 60-61, 66, 69, 76,
80, 93, 122-123, 150, 163, 165-
166, 169-170, 201-202, 204-205

L

Lateral collateral ligament (LCL)
15. *See also* LCL
LCL
15, 28, 29, 35, 40, 76, 81, 199-
200

ligament tears
34, 39-40, 59, 71, 77, 202

liniments
125

M

MacArthur Foundation
9
magnets
125-128

MCL
28-29, 35, 38, 40, 76, 81, 88,
199-200.

Medial Collateral Ligament
(MCL). *See* MCL
meniscus
14, 24-27, 36-37, 50, 55, 61, 64-67,
71, 76-79, 178, 188-189,
201, 202

methyl-sulfonyl-methane
(MSM). *See* MSM
minerals
97, 103, 114

MRI
45, 64-66, 68, 83, 188, 219

MSM
   109-111

N

nutrition
   107, 120, 243

O

orthotics
   18, 98-99

Osgood-Schlatter's disease
   53

osteochondritis dissecans
   56

osteochondroma
   53

P

patella. *See* kneecap

patellar tendinitis
   10, 34, 60, 69, 77, 87, 123, 143,
   147, 201-202, 204, 207

PCL
   15, 28-29, 35, 38, 40, 73-
   74, 76, 88, 199-200

physical therapy
   49, 124, 174

plica syndrome
   58

Posterior cruciate ligament
   15. *See also* PCL

R

rehabilitation
   17, 66, 75, 84, 86,
   87, 91, 116, 124, 155, 157, 159,
   161, 162, 174, 187, 189

running
   5, 9, 14, 25, 31, 38, 41-
   42, 45, 49, 51, 53, 61, 79, 91, 133,
   14, 162-163, 173, 198, 202-
   205, 207

S

search engines
   230-231

shark cartilage
   111

ski exercises
   136-152, 219-228

skiing
   9, 19, 124, 163, 171-173, 193,
   194-198, 201, 212, 214, 216-
   217

soccer
   38, 59, 80, 83, 147, 203, 216

sports medicine
   11, 14, 16-17, 47, 92, 237

sprains
   38-39, 81-85

Steadman, Richard Dr. 1

Steadman-Hawkins Clinic
   125, 143, 147, 207, 216, 222

strains
38-39, 81-85

support wraps
99

surgeon
knee replacement surgeries
11-12
considering surgery
145-147, 150, 152-153, 155,
160-163, 165-167, 171, 173-179
finding a surgeon
180-184, 186, 188-191, 204, 222,
229 *See also* doctor

surgery
4, 10-13, 15-16, 18, 19, 27, 40,
42, 49-50, 53, 58-60, 67-68,
76-77, 79, 81-83, 86, 88, 92-93,
107, 122-125, 135
considering surgery
145-150, 153, 156,
162, 165, 167, 171,
175, 177, 179,
finding a surgeon
180-181, 183-191, 193,
Internet research
232-233

swimming
9, 82-83, 96, 163, 207

T

tendinitis
34, 41, 49, 69, 76-77, 82, 123,
143, 207

tendon
5, 15, 17, 21-22, 29-31,
34-35, 41-42, 48-49, 51, 55,
60, 64-65, 69, 77, 80, 81,
83-84, 120, 123, 135, 143,

146-147, 151-153, 163, 200,
207, 215-216

tennis
9-10, 13, 19, 36, 60, 77, 79, 83,
87, 93, 148, 157, 163,
172-173, 194, 201-202, 204,
207, 216, 217

tibia
14-15, 22, 24, 26-29, 31, 34,
37, 39, 41, 45-47, 49, 51, 61,
64, 66, 71, 76, 78, 154-155,
163, 165-166, 168-69, 179, 189

torn cartilage
88

V

vitamins
106, 115-116

W

walking
17, 25, 37, 42, 76, 78, 87, 91, 93,
133, 157-158, 163, 171, 179,
202-203, 237

Web sites
orthopedic sites
236
general health sites
239
nutrition sites
243

X

X-ray
55, 67-71, 85, 88

Some Other New Harbinger Self-Help Titles

Virtual Addiction, $12.95
After the Breakup, $13.95
Why Can't I Be the Parent I Want to Be?, $12.95
The Secret Message of Shame, $13.95
The OCD Workbook, $18.95
Tapping Your Inner Strength, $13.95
Binge No More, $14.95
When to Forgive, $12.95
Practical Dreaming, $12.95
Healthy Baby, Toxic World, $15.95
Making Hope Happen, $14.95
I'll Take Care of You, $12.95
Survivor Guilt, $14.95
Children Changed by Trauma, $13.95
Understanding Your Child's Sexual Behavior, $12.95
The Self-Esteem Companion, $10.95
The Gay and Lesbian Self-Esteem Book, $13.95
Making the Big Move, $13.95
How to Survive and Thrive in an Empty Nest, $13.95
Living Well with a Hidden Disability, $15.95
Overcoming Repetitive Motion Injuries the Rossiter Way, $15.95
What to Tell the Kids About Your Divorce, $13.95
The Divorce Book, Second Edition, $15.95
Claiming Your Creative Self: True Stories from the Everyday Lives of Women, $15.95
Six Keys to Creating the Life You Desire, $19.95
Taking Control of TMJ, $13.95
What You Need to Know About Alzheimer's, $15.95
Winning Against Relapse: A Workbook of Action Plans for Recurring Health and Emotional Problems, $14.95
Facing 30: Women Talk About Constructing a Real Life and Other Scary Rites of Passage, $12.95
The Worry Control Workbook, $15.95
Wanting What You Have: A Self-Discovery Workbook, $18.95
When Perfect Isn't Good Enough: Strategies for Coping with Perfectionism, $13.95
Earning Your Own Respect: A Handbook of Personal Responsibility, $12.95
High on Stress: A Woman's Guide to Optimizing the Stress in Her Life, $13.95
Infidelity: A Survival Guide, $13.95
Stop Walking on Eggshells, $14.95
Consumer's Guide to Psychiatric Drugs, $16.95
The Fibromyalgia Advocate: Getting the Support You Need to Cope with Fibromyalgia and Myofascial Pain, $18.95
Healing Fear: New Approaches to Overcoming Anxiety, $16.95
Working Anger: Preventing and Resolving Conflict on the Job, $12.95
Sex Smart: How Your Childhood Shaped Your Sexual Life and What to Do About It, $14.95
You Can Free Yourself From Alcohol & Drugs, $13.95
Amongst Ourselves: A Self-Help Guide to Living with Dissociative Identity Disorder, $14.95
Healthy Living with Diabetes, $13.95
Dr. Carl Robinson's Basic Baby Care, $10.95
Better Boundries: Owning and Treasuring Your Life, $13.95
Goodbye Good Girl, $12.95
Fibromyalgia & Chronic Myofascial Pain Syndrome, $19.95
The Depression Workbook: Living With Depression and Manic Depression, $17.95
Self-Esteem, Second Edition, $13.95
Angry All the Time: An Emergency Guide to Anger Control, $12.95
When Anger Hurts, $13.95
Perimenopause, $16.95
The Relaxation & Stress Reduction Workbook, Fourth Edition, $17.95
The Anxiety & Phobia Workbook, Second Edition, $18.95
I Can't Get Over It, A Handbook for Trauma Survivors, Second Edition, $16.95
Messages: The Communication Skills Workbook, Second Edition, $15.95
Thoughts & Feelings, Second Edition, $18.95
Depression: How It Happens, How It's Healed, $14.95
The Deadly Diet, Second Edition, $14.95
The Power of Two, $15.95
Living Without Depression & Manic Depression: A Workbook for Maintaining Mood Stability, $18.95
Couple Skills: Making Your Relationship Work, $14.95
Hypnosis for Change: A Manual of Proven Techniques, Third Edition, $15.95
Letting Go of Anger: The 10 Most Common Anger Styles and What to Do About Them, $12.95
Infidelity: A Survival Guide, $13.95
When Anger Hurts Your Kids, $12.95
Don't Take It Personally, $12.95
The Addiction Workbook, $17.95

Call **toll free, 1-800-748-6273,** or log on to our online bookstore at **www.newharbinger.com** to order. Have your Visa or Mastercard number ready. Or send a check for the titles you want to New Harbinger Publications, Inc., 5674 Shattuck Ave., Oakland, CA 94609. Include $3.80 for the first book and 75¢ for each additional book, to cover shipping and handling. (California residents please include appropriate sales tax.) Allow two to five weeks for delivery.

Prices subject to change without notice.

Discount on the SportCord

The authors have secured for their readers a 10 percent discount from the manufacturers of the SportCord. Merely attach this coupon to your mail order to obtain your discount, or call and mention this ad in this book when you place your phone order.

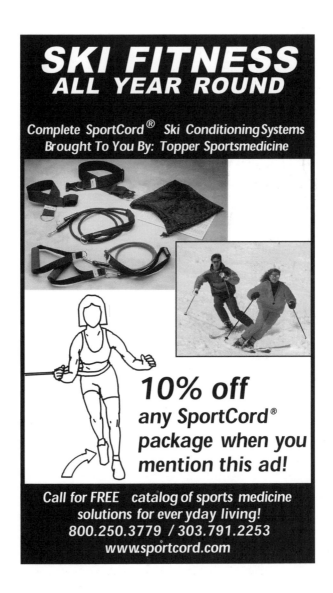

Questions for My Doctor